Air Fryer Cookbook:

100 Simple Delicious Recipes and Golden Tips to Success - Frying, Baking, Grilling and Roasting

I0425772

The trademarks that are used are without any consent, and the publication of the trademark is without permission or backing by the trademark owner. All trademarks and brands within this book are for clarifying purposes only and are the owned by the owners themselves, not affiliated with this document.

Table of Contents

Introduction

I want to thank you for choosing this book,*'Air Fryer Cookbook: 100 Simple Delicious Recipes and Golden Tips to Success - Frying, Baking, Grilling and Roasting.'*

Do you like French fries, onion rings or any other kind of fried foods? Well, who doesn't like fried food? If your answer is yes, then I am fairly certain that there might have been times when you felt a little guilty after munching on your favorite fried treats. The guilt quotient is certainly high when you are trying to stick to a diet or are trying to lose those extra pounds. Would you be excited if I told you that you now have the freedom to enjoy fried treats without the guilt that accompanies them? What if I told you that you could munch on fried foods without worrying about gaining a few extra pounds? Well, does this surprise you? There is a unique appliance that you can use to achieve all this and this appliance is an Air Fryer. Fried food that's cooked in an air fryer is not only healthy but isn't full of sinful calories. Does the idea of fried food being healthy confuse you? Well, hold on, this is a fact and not a myth! The Air Fryer is a wonderful kitchen appliance that allows you to cook all your favorite fried treats with little or even no oil.

The Air Fryer is a rather unique appliance that has revolutionized the world of cooking and frying in particular. You can always use a conventional deep fryer to fry foods, but this option isn't healthy. Instead of using oil or any other fat to fry foods, an Air Fryer uses hot air and hence its name.

An Air Fryer doesn't have to be restricted to just frying food! As you go through the recipes in this book, you will realize the truth embedded in this statement. You can enjoy crispy and crunchy fried foods that taste amazing without the added calories.

This book will help you realize that an Air Fryer is a truly amazing gift. If you like to eat home cooked food but don't have the time to cook or clean up, then the recipes given in this book will certainly come in handy. In this book, you will find 100 delicious and simple recipes that you can cook using an Air Fryer. These tried and tested recipes will help you whip up a nutritious and delicious feast by using only one appliance- the Air Fryer. An Air Fryer doesn't have to be used simply for cooking fries; you can cook so much more than just that.

So, if you are excited to start your journey into the world of healthy fried treats, then let us get started without further ado!

10 Best Air Fryers on Amazon

Please open the kindle version to click on the Air Fryers links below.

Get started with one of these top 10 Air Fryers on Amazon.com:

1. COSORI Air Fryers(100 Recipes included),3.7QT Electric Hot Air Fryer Oven Oilless Cooker,11 Cooking Presets,Preheat& Shake Reminder, LED One Touch Digital Screen,Nonstick Basket,2-Year Warranty,1500W

2. GoWISE USA 1700-Watt 5.8-QT 8-in-1 Digital Air Fryer and 50 Recipes for your Air Fryer Book (Black)

3. GoWISE USA 3.7-Quart Programmable Air Fryer with 8 Cook Presets, GW22638

4. Dash DFAF455GBAQ01 Deluxe Electric Air Fryer + Oven Cooker with Temperature Control, Non Stick Fry Basket, Recipe Guide + Auto Shut Off Feature 6 qt Aqua

5. Total Package XL Air Fryer, 100 Recipes Included, with Cooking Basket Divider and Deluxe Accessory Kit by Yedi Houseware (5.8 QT)

6. Air Fryer 5.5QT XL with ENKLOV 8 in 1 Digital Display Control,   Oil Less Airfryer Oven,1350W Electric Power Air Cooker,Come with Recipe Guide

7. Ultrean Air Fryer, 4.2Qt Electric Hot Air Fryers Oven Oilless Cooker with LCD Digital Screen and Easily Detachable Frying Pot, ETL/UL Certified,1-Year Warranty,1500W

8. OMORC Air Fryer XL, 5.8QT Air fryer (Recipe Guide Included) Electric Oven Oilless Cooker with Convenient Knob & Touch Screen, Nonstick Basket, 7 Cooking Presets, Preheat for Fast Healthier Fry Food

9. DmofwHi Large Air Fryer XL 8.5 QT, Digital Programmable Hot Air Fryer Toaster Oven 6 Preprogrammed Settings with Full Accessories, Viewing Window, Oilless Low-Fat Cooker

10. Secura Electric Hot Air Fryer Extra Large Capacity Air Fryer and additional accessories; Recipes and skewers accessory set (5.3Qt Sliver)

Golden Tips

1. Always preheat the air fryer for 5-8 minutes, unless specified otherwise.

2. If your air fryer has preset functions, you can use those functions like baking, grilling, frying, roasting etc.

3. Grease the air fryer basket, if using, with some cooking spray or rub some oil on the bottom and sides of the basket.

4. Preferably spray the food with some cooking spray. It is best to spray once half way through cooking. You need not spray on fatty food or greasy food.

5. Do not crowd the basket or cooking accessory. Preferably, place a single layer of the ingredients (it should not touch each other if you want it browned evenly all over) and cook in batches. This way the food cooks better and more evenly. In spite of not overcrowding, if your food is not crisping well enough then spray some more oil over it and continue cooking.

6. Always dry the food by patting with a clean kitchen towel or paper towels.

7. In case you are using some of your favorite oven recipes, set the temperature a few degrees less than you would have set your oven and also set the timer for a few minutes less than you would have set for your oven.

8. When you are frying smaller food pieces, pause the air fryer a couple of times and shake the food while cooking.

9. When you cook meat, it is best to check the temperature in the center of the meat to get an idea if the meat is cooked through or not. At times food looks nice and brown on the outside and turns out to be uncooked inside. So it is better to check the temperature.

10. At times you may notice smoke emanating from the air fryer unit. What you need to do right away is to switch off the air fryer and take out the air fryer basket. At times food may become embedded in the heating element, which can cause the smoke. In such a case, wait for the heating element to cool and clean it by wiping with a moist cloth.

11. At times when you are cooking oily food in the air fryer, you may discover white smoke coming out of the air fryer. This can be taken care of by adding 2-3 tablespoons of water in the bottom of the air fryer basket or placing a slice of bread. Bread will absorb the grease that is present. Bread is a good idea when bacon is being cooked, as it will absorb the fat released by bacon.

12. Be careful while cooking lightweight food, as it can flutter around with the speed of the fan of the air fryer. It can get stuck in the fan. So fasten the food with toothpicks. Food like tortillas, bread slices etc. can be fastened with toothpicks.

13. Always use good quality oil for spraying. Do not use aerosol spray cans.

14. It is a good idea to make slings from aluminum foil to lower the baking accessory inside the air fryer.

15. When the timer goes off, wait for a few seconds for the fan to turn off.

16. Place your air fryer on a heat resistant area and away from the wall by at least 5 inches.

17. Preferably use the accessories that come with the air fryer. If you do not have the accessories, then use ovenproof dishes and it should fit easily inside the air fryer basket.

18. Have an oil spray bottle for spraying over the food while using the air fryer. By drizzling oil over the food, you will end up using more oil.

19. To lower the accessories into the air fryer basket, make slings made of aluminum foil. Push the ends of the sling in the air fryer basket and then place the basket in the air fryer. This makes it easier to remove the dish later.

20. When you are breading any of the ingredients, shake to drop off excess bread. Press the bread that is already on the food so that it is slightly embedded in the food.

21. Once your food is cooked in the air fryer, first remove the air fryer basket from the air fryer before removing the food from the basket.

22. The cooked juices can be used to drizzle over the food if desired.

23. Clean the air fryer basket once you have finished operating the air fryer.

24. Once you have cleaned the air fryer basket and drawer, place it back in the air fryer. Switch on the air fryer for 2-3 minutes, which will dry the basket and drawer.
25. You can also reheat leftover food in the air fryer.

Chapter One: Air Fryer Chicken Recipes

Crispy Fried Chicken

Serves: 1-2

Ingredients:

- ½ cup all-purpose flour
- ½ teaspoon seasoning salt
- 2 chicken legs or thighs or breast, pat dried
- 2-3 teaspoons Old Bay Cajun seasoning
- 1 small egg
- Cooking spray

Method:

1. Add flour, Old Bay seasoning and seasoning salt into a shallow bowl. Stir until well combined.
2. Beat egg in a wide bowl.
3. Dredge chicken in the flour mixture. Next dip in the egg. Shake to drop off excess egg and finally dredge once more in the flour mixture.
4. Place chicken in the air fryer basket.
5. Air fry in a preheated air fryer at 380° F for 25 minutes.
6. Serve hot.

Tandoori Chicken Drummettes

Serves: 12

Ingredients:

- 1 dozen chicken drummettes, make a few slits all over the drummettes with a sharp knife

<u>For marinade:</u>

- 2 cloves garlic, peeled
- ¾ cup low fat yogurt
- ¼ inch piece ginger, peeled, chopped
- 1 teaspoon garam masala (Indian spice blend)
- 1 green chili
- ½ teaspoon salt or to taste
- A few drops orange food coloring (optional)
- Juice of a lemon
- 1 small onion, sliced + extra to serve
- A few lemon wedges to serve
- Spicy green chutney, to serve (optional)

Method:

1. Add ginger, garlic, green chili, onion, yogurt and garam masala into a blender. Blend for 30-40 seconds or until smooth.

2. Add lemon juice, salt and food coloring into a small bowl and mix well. Rub this over the chicken drummettes. Refrigerate for about 30 minutes.

3. Remove from the refrigerator and add the blended mixture over it, toss well.

4. Cover and refrigerate for 6-7 hours. Stir in between a couple of times while it is marinating.

5. Remove from the refrigerator an hour before cooking.

6. Place the chicken drummettes on the air fryer grill pan. Retain the marinade.

7. Place grill pan in the air fryer.

8. Grill in a preheated air fryer at 390° F for 10 minutes.

9. Brush the drummettes with the marinade. Spray a little cooking spray.

10. Air fry for another 3-4 minutes.

11. Serve with sliced onions and lemon wedges. Serve with green chutney if desired.

BBQ Chicken

Serves: 3

Ingredients:

- 1 whole chicken (about 2 ½ pounds), cut into thigh, breast and leg pieces
- ¾ teaspoon smoked paprika
- Salt to taste
- ¾ cup BBQ sauce
- ¾ teaspoon garlic powder

Method:

1. Sprinkle salt, garlic powder and paprika over the chicken pieces.
2. Lay the chicken pieces in the air fryer basket, with the skin side facing down.
3. Roast in a preheated air fryer at 375° F for 18 minutes. Air fry in batches if required.
4. Remove the chicken from the basket and place on a plate. Wipe the basket to remove any fat that may be settled on it.
5. Baste the chicken with BBQ sauce.
6. Place it in the air fryer basket, this time with the skin side facing up.
7. Lower the temperature to 350° F and roast for another 3-4 minutes.
8. Serve right away with some more BBQ sauce if desired.

General Tso Chicken

Serves: 2

Ingredients:

<u>For chicken:</u>

- ½ pound chicken thighs, skinless, boneless, chopped into chunks
- 3 tablespoons cornstarch
- Salt to taste
- White pepper to taste
- 1 small egg

<u>For Tso general sauce:</u>

- 1 teaspoon unseasoned rice wine vinegar
- 1 teaspoon corn starch
- 1 tablespoon soy sauce
- 1 teaspoon sugar
- 3 ½ tablespoons chicken stock or broth
- 1 tablespoon ketchup
- ½ tablespoon garlic, minced
- ½ tablespoon ginger, minced
- ½ teaspoon sesame oil
- 1-2 dried whole red chili, deseeded, chopped
- ½ teaspoon toasted sesame seeds
- 1 tablespoon thinly sliced green onion
- 1 teaspoon canola oil

Method:

1. To make chicken: Add egg into a bowl and beat well. Add chicken and stir.

2. Add cornstarch, salt and pepper into a shallow bowl and stir. Dredge the chicken in it. Shake the chicken to drop off excess cornstarch.

3. Preheat the air fryer for 3 minutes.

4. Place the chicken in the air fryer basket.

5. Air fry in a preheated air fryer at 400° F for 12-15 minutes or until brown and cooked through. Turn the chicken half way through cooking.

6. Meanwhile, make the Tso sauce as follows: Whisk together in a bowl, cornstarch, soy sauce, broth, sugar, ketchup and vinegar.

7. Place a pan over medium heat. Add canola oil into the pan and heat. Add chilies and stir for 4-5 seconds. Add ginger and garlic and sauté until aromatic. Add the cornstarch mixture and stir constantly until thick. Add chicken and heat thoroughly. Remove from heat.

8. Add ½ tablespoon green onion and sesame oil and stir.

9. Serve chicken over rice. Garnish with remaining green onion and sesame seeds and serve.

Roast Chicken

Serves: 6

Ingredients:

- 1 whole chicken of 3-3 ½ pounds
- Dry chicken rub or any other seasonings of your choice

Method:

1. Sprinkle dry rub liberally over the chicken. Rub it onto the chicken.
2. Lay the chicken in the air fryer basket, with the legs facing down.
3. Roast in a preheated air fryer at 330° F for 30 minutes.
4. Turn the chicken and roast for 15-20 minutes or the internal temperature shows 165° F.
5. Serve hot.

Chicken Drumsticks

Serves: 8

Ingredients:

- 8 chicken drumsticks, boneless
- 2 tablespoons mixed herbs
- ½ teaspoon black pepper powder
- 2 tablespoons honey or brown sugar
- ½ teaspoon salt or to taste
- ½ cup Dijon mustard
- 4 tablespoons olive oil

Method:

1. Add all the ingredients into a large bowl. Toss well. Cover and refrigerate for at least 5-6 hours. Toss the ingredients in between a couple of times.
2. Place an aluminum foil inside the air fryer basket. Place the chicken drumsticks inside the air fryer basket.
3. Bake in a preheated air fryer at 320° F for 10 minutes.
4. Increase the heat to 350° F and bake for 5-10 minutes or until skin is crisp.

Chicken Fillets with Brie and Cured Ham

Serves: 2

Ingredients:

- 1 large chicken fillet, halved
- 2 small slices Brie cheese or any other cheese of your choice
- 2 slices cured ham, halved
- ½ tablespoon finely chopped chives
- Freshly ground pepper to taste
- Salt to taste
- Olive oil, to brush

Method:

1. Slit the chicken fillet pieces horizontally, up to about ½ inch from the edges.
2. Sprinkle salt and pepper inside the fillet pieces.
3. Stuff a slice of Brie cheese and chives inside the slit of each piece.
4. Wrap each stuffed chicken piece with a slice (2 half pieces) of ham around it.
5. Brush with olive oil and place in the air fryer basket.
6. Roast in a preheated air fryer at 350° F for 15 minutes.
7. Turn the chicken pieces in between a couple of times.
8. Serve with mashed potatoes.

Crumbed Chicken Tenderloins

Serves: 2

Ingredients:

- ¼ cup dry breadcrumbs
- 4 chicken tenderloins
- 1 small egg, beaten
- 1 tablespoon vegetable oil

Method:

1. Preheat the air fryer for 18-20 minutes.
2. Add breadcrumbs and oil in a shallow bowl and mix well.
3. First drop the chicken in egg. Shake to drop off excess egg. Next dredge in the breadcrumbs and place in the air fryer basket.
4. Bake in a preheated air fryer at 350° F for 12-15 minutes. The internal temperature at the center of the meat should show 165° F.

Roasted Asian Chicken Wings

Serves: 2

Ingredients:

- 4 chicken wings, thawed
- 1 clove garlic, minced
- 1 teaspoon ground ginger
- ½ teaspoon ground cumin
- Freshly ground pepper to taste
- 3-4 tablespoons sweet chili sauce
- ¼ teaspoon salt or to taste

Method:

1. Mix together garlic, ginger, pepper, cumin and salt, in a bowl. Rub the chicken wings with this mixture.
2. Place the chicken wings in the air fryer basket. Spray with cooking spray.
3. Roast in a preheated air fryer at 350° F for 10 minutes or until brown.
4. Turn the chicken pieces half way through roasting.
5. Serve hot with sweet chili sauce.

Calzones

Serves: 4

Ingredients:

- 2 teaspoons olive oil
- 6 ounces baby spinach leaves
- 4 ounces shredded rotisserie chicken breast
- 3 ounces pre-shredded part-skim mozzarella cheese
- ½ cup minced red onion
- 2/3 cup marinara sauce
- 12 ounces fresh, prepared whole wheat pizza dough

Method:

1. Place a nonstick pan over medium-high heat. Add oil and heat. Add onion and sauté until translucent. Stir in the spinach and cook until it wilts. Turn off the heat.
2. Add marinara sauce and chicken and mix well.
3. Make 8 equal portions of the dough. Shape into balls.
4. Dust your countertop with a little flour. Roll the balls of dough into rounds of 6-inch diameter.
5. Divide the chicken mixture among the rolled dough and place it on one half of the circle. Fold the other half over the filling. The calzones are semi-circular now. Crimp the edges to seal the edges.
6. Spray calzones with cooking spray and place in the air fryer.

7. Bake in a preheated air fryer at 350° F for 12-15 minutes or until golden brown. Turn the calzones half way through baking.
8. Remove from the air fryer and cool for a few minutes.
9. Serve.

Sriracha Honey Chicken Wings

Serves: 1-2

Ingredients:

- ½ pound chicken wings, remove the tips and wings and cut into drummettes and flats
- 1 tablespoon sriracha sauce
- 2 tablespoons honey
- 2 teaspoons soy sauce
- Red pepper flakes to taste (optional if you want it spicier)
- ½ tablespoon butter
- Chopped cilantro, to garnish
- Sliced scallions, to garnish
- Chopped chives, to garnish
- 1 teaspoon lime juice or to taste

Method:

1. Place the chicken in the air fryer basket.
2. Air fry in a preheated air fryer at 360° F for about 30 minutes.
3. Turn the chicken 2-3 times while it is cooking.
4. Add sriracha sauce, honey, soy sauce, red pepper flakes and butter into a saucepan. Place saucepan over medium heat and simmer for 2-3 minutes.
5. Add chicken and toss until well coated.

6. Transfer into a bowl. Sprinkle lime juice, scallions, cilantro and chives and serve.

Panko Breaded Chicken Parmesan with Marinara Sauce

Serves: 4

Ingredients:

- 2 chicken breasts (8 ounces each) trimmed of fat, halved
- 4 tablespoons grated Parmesan cheese
- White of an egg, whisked
- 6 tablespoons low fat mozzarella cheese
- ½ cup panko breadcrumbs
- 1/3 - ½ cup marinara sauce
- Salt to taste
- Pepper to taste

Method:

1. Place chicken on the countertop. Pound with a meat mallet until flat.
2. Mix together in a shallow bowl breadcrumbs, salt, pepper and Parmesan cheese.
3. Dip the chicken in egg. Shake to drop off excess egg. Dredge the chicken in the breadcrumbs.
4. Spray some oil over it and place in the air fryer basket.
5. Bake in a preheated air fryer at 400° F for about 7 minutes.
6. Drizzle marinara sauce over it. Sprinkle mozzarella cheese on top.

7. Bake for a couple of minutes until the cheese melts.

Chicken Tikka

Serves: 2

For marinade:

- ¼ cup thick yogurt
- ½ teaspoon curry powder
- 2 teaspoons turmeric powder
- ¼ teaspoon smoked paprika
- 1 tablespoon ginger paste
- 1 tablespoon garlic paste
- 2 teaspoons salt
- ½ teaspoon garam masala powder (Indian spice blend)
- ½ tablespoon olive oil or any vegetable oil
- A few drops orange red food coloring (optional)

For chicken:

- ½ pound boneless chicken, cut into about 1 ½ inch pieces
- 1 medium onion, quartered, separate the layers of the onion
- 1 medium bell pepper, cut into 1 inch squares

To serve:

- 2 medium onions, sliced into rounds, separated into rings
- Lemon wedges
- 2 tablespoons fresh cilantro or mint leaves, chopped

Method:

1. Mix together all the ingredients for the marinade in a bowl and add chicken pieces to it. Mix until well coated.

2. Cover and refrigerate for at least 2 hours.

3. Remove from the refrigerator 30 minutes before frying.

4. Thread the chicken, onions and bell peppers on to skewers: - bell pepper-chicken- onion, in this manner. If using wooden skewers, soak in water for 30 minutes.

5. Place aluminum foil in the air fryer basket. Place skewers in the basket and the basket in the air fryer. Cook in batches.

8. Roast in a preheated air fryer at 400° F for about 15 minutes.

6. Turn the skewers in between a couple of times while roasting.

7. Remove the roasted chicken with onion and bell pepper on to a serving platter on a bed of onion rings. Garnish with cilantro and squeeze lemon juice over it.

8. Serve immediately.

Breakfast Burrito

Serves: 2

Ingredients:

- 6-8 slices chicken breast or turkey
- ½ red bell pepper, sliced
- ¼ cup mozzarella cheese, grated
- Salt to taste
- Pepper to taste
- 4 eggs
- ½ avocado, sliced
- 4 tablespoons salsa + extra to serve
- 2 tortillas

Method:

1. Spray the air-fryer baking accessory or use a small baking dish, which fits inside the air fryer with cooking spray.
2. Whisk eggs along with salt and pepper. Pour into the pan.
3. Place the pan in the air fryer.
4. Air fry at 390° F for 5 minutes. Remove the pan from the air fryer. Carefully remove the egg from the pan. Cut into strips.
5. Place aluminum foil in the air fryer tray.
6. Place the tortillas on your countertop. Place some egg strips, chicken slices, avocado, bell pepper and cheese over the tortillas. Spoon some salsa. Wrap and place on the prepared tray, with its seam side down.

7. Place the tray in the air fryer. Air fry at 350º F for 3 minutes or until cheese melts.

8. Serve hot with salsa as a dip.

BBQ Wontons

Serves: 10

Ingredients:

- 1 tablespoon grated zucchini
- 1 tablespoon grated carrot
- 1/8 cup chopped, cooked chicken
- 2 tablespoons cream cheese, softened
- 10 wonton wrappers
- ½ tablespoon pickled jalapeños, finely chopped
- 1 teaspoon BBQ sauce or to taste
- ½ tablespoon canola oil

Method:

1. Squeeze carrot and zucchini of excess moisture. Dry with paper towels.
2. Add zucchini, carrot, chicken, cream cheese, jalapeño and BBQ sauce into a bowl and mix well.
3. Place wonton wrappers on your countertop. Place about 2 teaspoons of the filling in the middle of every wonton wrapper. Run a finger dipped in water on the edges of each wrapper. Shape into wontons and seal the edges. Place on a plate and cover with a moist towel until you fry. Fry in batches.
4. Place the wontons in the baking accessory or a baking dish (grease with cooking spray) that can fit well into the air fryer.

5. Air fry in a preheated air fryer at 350° F for 4 minutes or until crisp and golden brown.

6. Remove the wontons and place on a wire rack for cool for a few minutes.

7. Serve with a dip of your choice or Sriracha sauce and serve.

Tandoori Chicken

Serves: 2

Ingredients:

<u>For chicken:</u>

- 4 chicken drumsticks, skinless, make 2-3 small slits on each drumstick
- A handful fresh cilantro, chopped, to garnish
- 2 teaspoons oil
- Lemon wedges, to serve
- Sliced onions, to serve

<u>For marinade:</u>

- 1 cup plain Greek yogurt
- 1 teaspoon chili powder
- 1 teaspoon salt or to taste
- ½ teaspoon ground cumin
- ½ teaspoon ground coriander
- ½ teaspoon turmeric powder
- 2 tablespoons lemon juice
- Lemon wedges to serve
- 2 teaspoons ginger paste
- 2 teaspoons garlic paste
- ½ tablespoon dried fenugreek leaves

Method:

1. Place yogurt in a fine wire mesh strainer. Place strainer over a bowl and let it drain for 4-5 hours. Alternately, place it in cheesecloth. Tie it up and hang it for a few hours to drop off excess moisture from the yogurt. Place a bowl below the cheesecloth to collect the dropped liquid. Transfer drained yogurt into a large bowl.

2. Add rest of the ingredients for marinade except lemon wedges and cilantro. Mix well. Add chicken and stir until well coated.

3. Cover and refrigerate for 6-7 hours. Turn the chicken in between a couple of times.

4. Remove from the refrigerator about an hour before frying.

5. Place an aluminum foil in the air fryer basket. Place the chicken pieces in the basket and spray with cooking spray. Place the basket in the air fryer.

6. Grill in a preheated air fryer at 360° F for 15 minutes or until brown. Turn the chicken pieces in between a couple of times. Spray some cooking spray after turning the chicken.

7. Serve chicken garnished with cilantro and with lemon wedges and onion slices.

Turkish Bread with Chicken Filling

Serves: 4

Ingredients:

<u>For filling:</u>

- 2 pounds chicken fillet, cut into strips
- 4 red onions, cut into rings
- 2 Turkish breads
- 4 tomatoes, sliced
- 2 teaspoons smoked paprika powder
- ¼ teaspoon chili powder
- 4 tablespoons olive oil
- 2 teaspoons cumin powder
- Salt to taste
- Pepper powder to taste
- Rocket lettuce leaves to serve

<u>For sauce:</u>

- 2 cups 0% fat, Turkish yogurt
- 2 tablespoons chopped parsley
- 6 cloves garlic, minced and then crushed

Method:

1. Add oil, chili powder, paprika, cumin, salt and pepper into a bowl and stir. Add chicken strips to it. Toss well and marinate for an hour.

2. Meanwhile, make the sauce as follows: Mix together all the ingredients of the sauce in a bowl. Cover and set aside for a while for the flavors to set in.

3. Place only the chicken strips in the air fryer basket, discarding the marinade.

4. Air fry in a preheated air fryer at 390° F for 10 minutes.

5. Cut each of the Turkish breads into 4 pieces.

6. Fill the chicken strips, onions and tomatoes inside the Turkish bread. Drizzle some sauce as well.

7. Serve over rocket lettuce.

Southern Fried Chicken

Serves: 3

Ingredients:

For chicken:

- 3 chicken legs (about a pound)
- ½ cup self-rising flour
- 1 egg, at room temperature
- 1 tablespoon milk or buttermilk
- Olive oil, as required
- 2 tablespoons cornstarch
- ½ tablespoon hot sauce
- 2 tablespoons water

For spice mix:

- 1 teaspoon pepper
- 1 teaspoon paprika
- ½ -¾ teaspoon Italian seasoning
- 1 teaspoon sea salt
- ¾ teaspoon garlic powder
- ½ teaspoon onion powder

Method:

1. Add all the ingredients for spice mix into a bowl and stir.

2. Sprinkle half of the spice mixture over the chicken. Drizzle some oil if required. Rub the mixture well onto the chicken pieces.

3. Add cornstarch, flour and remaining spice mix into a shallow bowl and stir until well combined. Taste and add more of the spice mix and salt if required. It is necessary that the flour mixture should be nice and spicy with adequate salt in it.

4. Add egg, milk, hot sauce and water into a bowl and whisk well.

5. Lightly dredge the chicken pieces in the flour mixture. Shake to drop off excess flour mixture. Place on a baking sheet for 10 minutes.

6. Dip the chicken in the egg mixture. Shake to drop off excess egg.

7. Next dredge in the flour mixture once again. Shake to drop off excess flour mixture.

8. Place on the baking sheet for 10-12 minutes.

9. Brush some oil over the chicken. Place in the air fryer basket.

10. Air fry in a preheated air fryer at 350° F for 18 minutes.

11. Flip sides half way through frying. Brush some more oil over the chicken if required.

12. Take out the chicken from the basket and let it sit for 5 minutes before serving.

Zinger Chicken Burger

Serves: 2

Ingredients:

- 3 chicken breasts
- 2 tablespoons plain flour
- 2 ounces breadcrumbs
- ½ teaspoon mustard powder
- Salt to taste
- Pepper to taste
- 1 very small egg beaten (or beat an egg and use half of it)
- 2-3 teaspoons KFC spice blend
- ½ teaspoon Worcestershire sauce
- ½ teaspoon paprika

For KFC spice blend:

- 1 teaspoon salt
- 1 teaspoon dried oregano
- ½ tablespoon black pepper
- 2 tablespoons paprika
- ½ tablespoon ground ginger
- 1 teaspoon dried oregano
- 1 teaspoon dried basil
- ½ tablespoon celery salt
- ½ tablespoon dried mustard
- 1 tablespoon garlic salt

- 1 ½ tablespoons white pepper

Method:

1. To make KFC spice blend: Add all the ingredients for KFC spice blend into a small jar and stir until well combined. Use as much as required. Fasten the lid of the jar and store the remaining for future use.

2. To make chicken: Add chicken into the food processor bowl. Process until well minced.

3. Add Worcestershire sauce, salt, pepper, paprika and mustard and process until well combined.

4. Transfer into a bowl. Divide the mixture into 2 equal portions and shape into burgers.

5. Beat egg in a bowl. Place flour on a plate. Add breadcrumbs and KFC spice mix into another bowl.

6. First dredge burgers in flour. Shake to drop off excess flour. Next dip in egg. Shake to drop off excess egg and finally dredge in the breadcrumb mixture.

7. Place in the air fryer basket.

8. Air fry in a preheated air fryer at 350° F for 15 minutes or until cooked through.

Pizza Stuffed Chicken

Serves: 2

Ingredients:

- 4 chicken thighs, skinless, boneless
- 12 slices turkey pepperoni
- 4 ounces mozzarella cheese, sliced
- 6-7 tablespoons pizza sauce
- 1 small red onion, sliced
- 2/3 cup shredded cheese

Method:

1. Unfold the chicken thighs and place them flat on a sheet of parchment paper.
2. Place another sheet of parchment paper over the chicken and pound with a meat mallet until thin. Remove the top sheet of parchment paper.
3. Spread pizza sauce over the chicken. Lay 3 slices of pepperoni on each chicken. Place a cheese slice over the pepperoni. Fold the chicken like you would close a book.
4. Fasten with toothpicks. Carefully lift and place on a greased baking tray of the air fryer.
5. Preheat the air fryer for 2 minutes.
6. Place baking tray in the air fryer.
7. Bake at 370° F for 12 minutes or until chicken is cooked. Flip sides half way through baking.

8. Place remaining cheese slices on top during the final 3 minutes of cooking.

Chicken Pot Pie

Serves: 2

Ingredients:

- 4 chicken tenders
- 1 potato, peeled, diced
- 1 bay leaf
- Yolk of 1 egg
- Refrigerated buttermilk dough for 4 biscuits
- 1 ¼ cups condensed cream of celery soup
- 2/3 cup heavy cream
- 1 sprig thyme
- 2 teaspoons milk

Method:

1. Add chicken, potato, bay leaf, soup, heavy cream and thyme into a saucepan.
2. Place the saucepan over medium heat. When it begins to boil, turn off the heat.
3. Transfer into the baking accessory or a baking pan that can fit well into the air fryer.
4. Cover the dish with foil and place in the air fryer.
5. Bake in a preheated air fryer at 320° F for about 15 minutes.
6. Whisk together egg yolk and milk in a bowl.
7. Place biscuits on top of the chicken mixture in the baking dish. Brush egg mixture over the biscuits.

8. Lower the temperature of the air fryer to 300° F. Bake for another 10 minutes or until the biscuits are golden brown in color.

9. Remove from the air fryer and cool for 4-5 minutes before serving.

Baked Thai Peanut Chicken Egg Rolls

Serves: 2

Ingredients:

- 2 egg roll wrappers
- 2 tablespoons Thai peanut sauce
- 2 green onions, chopped
- 1 cup shredded rotisserie chicken
- 1 small carrot, very thinly sliced
- 1/8 red bell pepper, julienned

Method:

1. Place chicken in a bowl. Drizzle Thai peanut sauce over it and stir until well combined.
2. Place the egg roll wrappers on your countertop. Divide equally and place carrot, onion and bell pepper on the bottom third of the wrappers. Divide the chicken and place over the vegetables.
3. Brush the edges of the wrappers with water. Fold the sides slightly over the filling and then roll the wrappers tightly. Cover with moist paper towels until ready to fry.
4. Spray the egg rolls all over, with cooking spray. Place in the air fryer basket.
5. Air fry in a preheated air fryer at 390° F for 6-8 minutes or until crisp.
6. Remove from the air fryer and place on your cutting board.

7. Cut into 2 halves and serve with some more Thai peanut sauce.

Pecan Chicken Salad Sandwiches

Serves: 2

Ingredients:

- ½ pound chicken breast
- A handful red grapes, diced
- 1 stalk celery, chopped
- ¼ cup mayonnaise
- Romaine lettuce leaves, as required
- 1 small avocado, peeled, pitted, sliced
- Salt to taste
- Pepper to taste
- 1 small apple, peeled, cored, chopped
- 2 tablespoons chopped pecans
- ¼ teaspoon sea salt or to taste
- 4 slices honey wheat bread or your favorite bread

Method:

1. Sprinkle salt and pepper over the chicken and place in the air fryer basket.
2. Air fry in a preheated air fryer at 340° F for 15 minutes or until cooked through.
3. Remove from the air fryer and place on your cutting board.
4. When cool enough to handle, chop the chicken into bite size cubes and place in a bowl.

5. Add celery, grapes, pecans and apples and mayonnaise and fold gently.

6. Cover and chill for an hour.

7. Toast the bread slices. Top the salad over 2 slices of bread. Place avocado slices and cover the sandwiches with the remaining 2 slices of bread.

Hot Chicken Salad

Serves: 2

Ingredients:

- ½ pound chicken breast
- 2 shallots, chopped
- 2 stalks celery, chopped
- ½ cup cream cheese
- 2 tablespoons chopped chives
- ½ teaspoon onion powder
- ½ teaspoon garlic powder
- Freshly cracked pepper to taste
- ½ cup shredded cheddar cheese
- Salt to taste

Method:

1. Sprinkle salt and pepper over the chicken and place in the air fryer basket.
2. Air fry in a preheated air fryer at 340° F for 15 minutes or until cooked through.
3. Remove from the air fryer and place on your cutting board.
4. When cool enough to handle, chop the chicken into bite size cubes or shred the chicken.

5. Add all the ingredients except about ¼ of cheddar cheese and chicken into the baking accessory or a small baking dish that fits well into the air fryer.

6. Stir until well combined. Add chicken and stir until well combined.

7. Sprinkle ¼ cup cheddar cheese over the salad.

8. Bake for 3-4 minutes until cheese melts.

Crispy Cheesy Chicken

Serves: 4

Ingredients:

- 2 thin chicken breasts
- 7-8 tablespoons shaved Parmesan-Asiago cheese blend
- Freshly ground pepper to taste
- 4 tablespoons panko breadcrumbs
- Salt to taste
- ½ cup milk

Method:

1. Add salt, pepper and milk into a bowl and stir. Place chicken in this mixture for 10 minutes.
2. Mix together in a bowl breadcrumbs and Parmesan cheese blend.
3. Remove the chicken from the milk mixture. Shake to drop off excess milk. Dredge the chicken in the breadcrumbs mixture and place in the air fryer basket. Cook in batches if required.
4. Spray some oil on top.
5. Air fry in a preheated air fryer at 350° F for about 15-16 minutes. Flip sides after 8 minutes of frying. Spray some oil on top.

Chapter Two: Air Fryer Beef Recipes

Air Fryer Steak

Serves: 2

Ingredients:

- 2 New York strip steak or Rib eye steak
- Salt to taste
- Paprika to taste
- Pepper to taste
- 1 teaspoon garlic powder or to taste
- Butter, to serve

Method:

1. Spray the steak all over, with olive oil spray.
2. Sprinkle salt, paprika, garlic powder and pepper over it.
3. Grill in a preheated air fryer to 400° F for 12 minutes or until the desired doneness. Flip sides half way through frying.
4. Serve with butter.

Herbed Roast Beef and Potatoes

Serves: 4-6

Ingredients:

- 2 pounds top round roast beef
- Freshly ground pepper to taste
- ½ teaspoon salt
- ½ teaspoon minced, fresh rosemary
- ½ teaspoon dried thyme
- 1-½ pounds red potatoes, chopped into bite-sized pieces.
- 1 tablespoon olive oil

Method:

1. Mix together all the ingredients except beef and potatoes in a bowl.
2. Rub 1-teaspoon oil all over the beef. Rub the herb mixture all over the beef.
3. Place an aluminum foil at the bottom of the air fryer basket.
4. Place roast in the air fryer basket.
5. Bake in a preheated air fryer at 360° F for about 18 minutes. Flip sides of the roast.
6. Add potatoes into a bowl. Drizzle remaining oil over it. Season with salt and pepper and toss well.

7. Place the potatoes around the roast. Roast for 20 minutes or until potatoes are cooked. Turn the roast and potatoes a couple of times while roasting.

8. Remove roast from the air fryer and place on your cutting board. When cool enough to handle, slice the roast and serve potatoes and with a gravy or sauce of your choice, if desired.

Juicy Cheeseburgers

Serves: 2

Ingredients:

- ½ pound ground chuck beef
- ½ teaspoon Worcestershire sauce
- Salt to taste
- Pepper to taste
- 2 burger buns, split, lightly toast if desired
- 2 slices cheese
- ½ teaspoon liquid smoke
- 2 teaspoons burger seasoning
- Mayonnaise if desired
- Toppings of your choice like lettuce, tomato slices etc. (optional)

Method:

1. Add beef, seasoning, salt, pepper, Worcestershire sauce and liquid smoke into a bowl and mix until well combined.
2. Divide the mixture into 2 equal portions and shape into patties.
3. Place in the air fryer basket.

4. Grill in a preheated air fryer to 360° F for 12 minutes or until the desired doneness. Flip sides half way through frying.
5. Place a slice of cheese over each burger.
6. Place in the air fryer. Grill for a minute or until cheese melts.
7. Place a burger on each of the bottom half of the buns. Apply mayonnaise on the cut part of the buns if desired. Place toppings if using. Cover with the top half of the buns and serve.

Meat Croquettes

Serves: 4

Ingredients:

- 1 small onion, finely chopped
- 7 ounces veal or beef, finely chopped
- 4 tablespoons butter
- Salt to taste
- Pepper powder to taste
- ¼ teaspoon ground nutmeg
- 1 cup almond milk or soy milk, unsweetened
- 3 tablespoons flour
- 2 tablespoons vegetable oil
- ½ cup breadcrumbs

Method:

1. Place a skillet over medium heat. Add butter. When butter melts, add onions and meat and sauté for a few seconds. Add flour and sauté for few seconds until fragrant.
2. Pour milk slowly, stirring simultaneously. Cook until thick. Add salt, pepper and nutmeg and mix well. Turn off the heat. Cool completely. Chill for 2 hours.
3. Add breadcrumbs and oil into a bowl and mix until crumbly.

4. Remove from meat mixture from the refrigerator and shape into croquettes.

5. Roll in breadcrumbs and place in the air fryer basket.

6. Bake in a preheated air fryer at 390° F for about 8-10 minutes or until golden brown. Turn the croquettes half way through frying.

7. Serve with ketchup or dip of your choice.

Italian Meatballs

Serves: 6

Ingredients:

- 1 tablespoon olive oil
- ½ tablespoon minced garlic
- 1 tablespoon whole milk
- 2 1/3 ounces bulk turkey sausage
- 5 1/3 ounces lean, ground beef
- 1 small egg, lightly beaten
- ½ tablespoon minced fresh rosemary
- 2 tablespoons minced fresh flat-leaf parsley
- ½ tablespoon minced fresh thyme
- ¼ teaspoon kosher salt or to taste
- 1 small shallot, minced
- 2 tablespoons whole wheat panko breadcrumbs
- ½ tablespoon Dijon mustard

Method:

1. Place a nonstick pan over medium heat. Add oil and heat. Add shallot and sauté until translucent.
2. Stir in the garlic and sauté until aromatic. Turn off the heat.
3. Add milk and breadcrumbs into a bowl and stir. Let it soak for 5 minutes.

4. Add shallot mixture, beef, sausage, herbs, salt, egg and mustard into the bowl of breadcrumbs and mix well.

5. Divide the mixture into 12 equal portions and shape into balls.

6. Place in the air fryer basket.

7. Bake in a preheated air fryer at 400° F for about 10-12 minutes or until light brown and cooked through. Turn the meatballs half way through baking.

8. Serve as it is for a snack or with pasta or rice along with some sauce as main course.

Courgette Stuffed with Meat

Serves: 4

Ingredients:

- 2 large courgettes, trimmed
- 2 cloves garlic, crushed
- 14 ounces lean ground beef
- ½ cup feta cheese, crumbled
- 1 tablespoon mild paprika powder
- Freshly ground pepper to taste
- Salt to taste

Method:

1. Slice off the ends of the courgettes. Slice each courgette into 6 equal rounds.
2. Scoop out the flesh with a teaspoon leaving about ½ inch from the bottom and ¼ inch from the sides. So you have courgette cases that are hollow inside.
3. Sprinkle salt inside the courgettes.
4. Add rest of the ingredients into a bowl. Divide this mixture into 12 equal portions and stuff the mixture into the courgette cases. Press well.
5. Cook the courgettes in batches.

6. Place a few courgette slices in the air fryer basket.

7. Bake in a preheated air fryer at 350° F for about 10-12 minutes.

8. Serve hot with cherry tomatoes and rice to complete a meal.

Taco Bell Crunch Wraps

Serves: 3

Ingredients:

- 1 pound ground beef
- 2/3 cup water
- 2 small Roma tomatoes
- 1 cup shredded lettuce
- 1 cup sour cream
- Taco seasoning to taste
- 3 flour tortillas (12 inches each)
- 6 ounces nacho cheese
- 1 cup Mexican blend cheese
- 3 tostadas

Method:

1. Place a skillet over medium heat. Add beef and cook until brown. Turn off the heat. Drain the fat remaining in the pan.
2. Add taco seasoning and mix well. Cook for a couple of minutes. Turn off the heat.
3. Spread the tortillas on your countertop. Divide the beef among the tortillas.

4. Sprinkle the nacho cheese over the meat. Place a tostada on each. Divide the sour cream, lettuce, tomatoes and cheese equally and place over the nacho cheese layer.

5. Wrap tightly and place in the air fryer basket, with the seam side facing down.

6. Spray the wraps with cooking spray. Fry in batches.

7. Air fry in a preheated air fryer at 350° F for about 2 minutes. Flip sides and fry for 2 minutes.

8. Remove from the air fryer and cool for a couple of minutes before serving.

Korean BBQ Beef

Serves: 2

Ingredients:

<u>For meat:</u>

- 2 tablespoons cornstarch
- ½ pound thinly sliced flank steak or thinly sliced steak

<u>For sauce:</u>

- ¼ cup soy sauce
- 1 tablespoon white wine vinegar
- ½ tablespoon hot chili sauce
- ¼ teaspoon sesame seeds
- ½ tablespoon water
- ¼ cup brown sugar
- 1 small clove garlic, crushed
- ½ teaspoon ground ginger
- ½ tablespoon cornstarch

<u>To serve:</u>

- Green onion, sliced
- Green beans
- Cooked rice

Method:

1. Place a sheet of aluminum foil in the air fryer basket. Spray with cooking spray, preferably coconut oil spray.
2. Place steak in the basket. Spray the steak with cooking spray.
3. Air fry in a preheated air fryer at 350° F for about 2 minutes. Flip sides and fry for 2 minutes.
4. Meanwhile, mix together water and cornstarch in a bowl. Set aside. Add rest of the sauce ingredients into a saucepan. Place saucepan over medium heat. When it begins to boil, add cornstarch mixture and stir constantly until the sauce thickens.
5. Place steak slices on a serving platter. Pour sauce on top.
6. Serve with the suggested serving options.

Meat Loaf

Serves: 8

Ingredients:

- 1 ¾ pounds lean ground beef
- 6 tablespoons whole wheat breadcrumbs
- 1 medium onion, finely chopped
- 2 teaspoons freshly ground black pepper powder
- Salt to taste
- 2 eggs, lightly beaten

- 3 1/2 ounces salami or chorizo sausage, finely chopped
- 4 mushrooms, cut into thick slices
- 2 tablespoons fresh thyme
- A little olive oil to brush

Method:

1. Add all the ingredients except mushrooms into a bowl. Mix with your hands until well combined.
2. Transfer the mixture into the bread pan or baking accessory of the air fryer. Spread the mixture evenly and smoothly.
3. Place mushroom slices on top of the meat and press it slightly into the meat.
4. Brush the top with olive oil.
5. Bake in a preheated air fryer at 390º F for about 25 minutes or until brown.
6. Remove from the air fryer and let it rest for 10-12 minutes.
7. Slice into wedges and serve with a salad of your choice and fried potatoes.

Carne Asada

Serves: 2

Ingredients:

- 1 medium onion, thinly sliced
- 1 pound skirt steak about ½-1 inch thick

For marinade:

- 2-3 whole chipotle peppers in adobo
- ¼ cup fresh orange juice
- 2 tablespoon fresh lemon juice
- 2 tablespoons fresh lime juice
- 1 pasilla pepper, roasted, peeled, chopped
- 3 cloves garlic, peeled
- ½ cup chopped cilantro
- ½ tablespoon kosher salt
- 1 teaspoon dried oregano
- 1 tablespoon extra-virgin olive oil
- 1 tablespoon light brown sugar
- 1 teaspoon ground cumin
- ½ teaspoon freshly ground pepper

To serve:

- Tortillas

- Shredded cabbage
- Avocado slices
- Lime wedges
- Cilantro

Method:

1. Add all the ingredients for marinade into the food processor bowl. Blend until smooth.
2. Retain 3-4 tablespoons of the marinade to serve as dip.
3. Pour remaining marinade into a bowl. Add onion and steak and mix well. Cover and chill for 3-8 hours.
4. Preheat the air fryer for 10 minutes. Place steak and onion (without marinade)
5. Grill in a preheated air fryer at 400° F for about 6-10 minutes, until the desired doneness.
6. Remove steak from the air fryer and place on your cutting board. When cool enough to handle, thinly slice the steak against the grain.
7. Place tortillas on your countertop. Place steak slices over it. Top with cabbage, avocado and cilantro.
8. Wrap and serve with lemon wedges and retained dip.

Fried Meatballs in Tomato Sauce

Serves: 6

Ingredients:

- 1 ½ pounds ground beef
- 1 tablespoons fresh thyme, chopped
- 2 tablespoons fresh parsley, chopped
- 1 large onion, minced
- 1/3 cup whole wheat breadcrumbs
- 2 eggs
- Salt to taste
- Pepper to taste
- 2 cups tomato sauce of your choice
- Cooked spaghetti to serve

Method:

1. Add all the ingredients except tomato sauce into a large bowl. Mix until well combined.
2. Make small balls of the mixture of about 1 - 1-½ inch diameter.
3. Place the balls in the air fryer basket.
4. Bake in a preheated air fryer at 390⁰ F for 7 minutes. Fry the meatballs in batches if required.

5. When done, transfer the balls in the baking accessory or a baking dish that is smaller than the air fryer and fits well inside the air fryer.
6. Pour tomato sauce over it and stir. Place the dish in the air fryer basket.
7. Reduce the temperature to 330° F and cook for another 5 minutes.
8. Serve over cooked spaghetti.

Beef Satay

Serves: 4

Ingredients:

- 2 pounds flank steak, thinly sliced into long strips
- 2 tablespoons fish sauce
- 2 tablespoons minced ginger
- 2 tablespoons sugar
- 2 teaspoons ground coriander
- ½ cup chopped, roasted peanuts, to garnish
- 4 tablespoons oil
- 2 tablespoons soy sauce
- 2 tablespoons minced garlic
- 2 teaspoons Sriracha sauce or hot sauce of your choice
- ½ cup chopped cilantro + extra to serve

Method:

1. Add all the ingredients except peanuts into a large bowl and mix well.
2. Chill for 1-8 hours.
3. Remove the beef strips with a pair of tongs. Shake to drop off excess marinade and place in the air fryer basket. Do not overlap. Discard the marinade.
4. Grill in a preheated air fryer at 400° F for about 8 minutes. Flip sides once half way through grilling.

5. Garnish with cilantro and roasted peanuts. Serve with peanut sauce if desired.

Steak Tacos

Serves: 3

Ingredients:

- ½ pound skirt steak
- Pepper to taste
- Salt to taste
- ¼ teaspoon garlic powder
- ½ cup shredded red cabbage
- 3 corn tortillas
- 4-5 teaspoons sour cream
- 6 tablespoons shredded Monterey Jack cheese

For avocado salsa:

- ½ avocado, peeled, pitted, finely chopped
- 2 teaspoons minced white onion
- Fresh lime juice, to taste
- 1 small tomato, finely chopped
- Salt to taste

Method:

1. To make avocado salsa: Add all the ingredients for avocado salsa into a bowl and mix well. Cover and set aside for a while for the flavors to set in.
2. Sprinkle salt, pepper and garlic powder all over the steak.

82

3. Place in the air fryer basket.

4. Grill in a preheated air fryer at 400° F for about 10 minutes. Flip sides once half way through grilling.

5. Remove steak and place on your cutting board. When cool enough to handle, slice the steak.

6. Place tortillas on your countertop. Spread sour cream on each tortilla. Scatter some red cabbage over it. Divide the steak slices among the tortillas and place over the cabbage.

7. Sprinkle cheese on top.

8. Wrap and serve with avocado salsa.

Schnitzel Parmigiana

Serves: 2

Ingredients:

- 2 pre-crumbed beef schnitzel
- ½ cup grated Parmesan cheese
- 1/3-1/2 cup pasta sauce of your choice

Method:

1. Place the schnitzel in the air fryer basket.
2. Air fry in a preheated air fryer at 350 º F for 15 minutes. Remove from the air fryer and place in the baking accessory.
3. Pour pasta sauce over the schnitzel.
4. Sprinkle cheese all over it.
5. Air fry for another 5 minutes or until the cheese melts.
6. Serve hot.

Beef Stir Fry with Marinade

Serves: 2-3

Ingredients:

- ½ pound beef sirloin, cut into 2 inch strips
- ½ red bell pepper, cut into strips
- ½ yellow bell pepper, cut into strips
- ½ green bell pepper, cut into strips
- ¾ pound broccoli, cut into florets
- 1 small onion, thinly sliced
- 1 small red onion, thinly sliced
- ½ tablespoon vegetable oil

For marinade:

- 2 tablespoons hoisin sauce
- ½ teaspoon sesame oil
- ½ teaspoon ground ginger
- 1 teaspoon minced garlic
- ½ tablespoon soy sauce
- 2 tablespoons water

Method:

1. Mix together all the ingredients for sauce into a bowl.
2. Stir in the meat. Cover and chill for 20-30 minutes.

3. Add all the vegetables into a bowl. Drizzle oil over it and toss well. Transfer into the air fryer basket.

4. Air fry in a preheated air fryer at 390 º F for 5 minutes or until tender.

5. Transfer into a bowl.

6. Place beef in the air fryer basket.

7. Air fry in a preheated air fryer at 360 º F for 6 minutes. Flip sides half way through frying.

8. Serve over rice. Place vegetables over the meat and serve.

Corned Beef and Cabbage Egg Rolls

Serves: 3

Ingredients:

- 6 ounces corned beef, shredded
- 6 egg roll wrappers
- ¾ cup stewed cabbage
- Spicy mustard to serve

Method:

1. Place an egg roll wrapper on your countertop in such a manner that one of the corners is facing you.
2. Place about 2 tablespoons of corned beef, diagonally, from one corner to the other, but do not fill in the corners. Place a tablespoon of cabbage on the corned beef.
3. Now fold the corners over the filling to seal it. Fold the sides and roll to create a log. Brush the edges with water and press to seal.
4. Fill the remaining wrappers similarly.
5. Spray the egg rolls all over with cooking spray. Place the rolls in the air fryer basket.
6. Air fry in a preheated air fryer at 400 º F or about 7 minutes or until golden brown.

7. Remove from the air fryer and cool for a few minutes before serving.

8. Dip in spicy mustard and enjoy.

Roasted Stuffed Peppers

Serves: 4

Ingredients:

- 4 medium green bell peppers, halved lengthwise, deseeded, de-stemmed
- 2 cloves garlic, minced
- 1 pound lean ground beef
- 2 teaspoons Worcestershire sauce
- Pepper to taste
- 8 ounces cheddar cheese, shredded
- 1 medium onion, chopped
- 2 teaspoons olive oil
- 1 cup tomato sauce
- Salt to taste

Method:

1. Place a saucepan with water over medium heat. Bring to a boil. Add bell pepper and cook for 2 minutes. Drain the water and pat the peppers dry with paper towels.
2. Place a pan over medium heat. Add oil and heat. Add onion and garlic and sauté until golden brown in color. Turn off the heat.

3. Transfer into a mixing bowl. Add beef, Worcestershire sauce, half the cheese, pepper, salt and ½ cup tomato sauce and mix until well combined.

4. Fill this mixture into the bell pepper halves. Spread remaining sauce on each. Sprinkle cheese on top.

5. Place in the baking accessory of the air fryer or a small baking dish that can fit well into the air fryer.

6. Roast in a preheated air fryer at 390 $^{\circ}$ F or about 15-17 minutes or until meat is cooked.

7. Remove from the air fryer and cool for a few minutes before serving.

Saltimbocca Veal rolls with Sage

Serves: 2

Ingredients:

- ¾ cup meat stock
- 2 veal cutlets
- 4 fresh sage leaves
- 1 ½ tablespoons butter, softened
- 1/3 cup dry white wine
- 2 slices cured ham
- Freshly ground pepper to taste
- Salt to taste

Method:

1. To make gravy: Add stock and wine in a saucepan and place the saucepan over medium heat. Bring to a boil. Continue boiling until the liquid is reduced to about 1/3 the original quantity. Turn off the heat and transfer into a bowl. Keep warm.
2. Season the cutlets with salt and pepper. Cover the cutlets with sage leaves.
3. Roll the cutlets tightly and wrap a ham slice around each cutlet. Brush the cutlets lightly with butter.
4. Place the rolled cutlets in the air fryer basket.

5. Roast in a preheated air fryer at 390 º F or about 10 minutes.

6. Reduce the temperature to 300 º F and cook for 5 minute more. When done, remove cutlets from the basket and place on your cutting board.

7. When cool enough to handle, slice the veal rolls.

8. Add the remaining butter to the reduced stock and wine mixture. Add salt and pepper.

9. Serve sliced veal rolls with gravy.

Mongolian Beef

Serves: 2-3

Ingredients:

<u>For meat:</u>

- 2 tablespoons cornstarch
- ½ pound flank steak, thinly sliced lengthwise

<u>For sauce:</u>

- 1 teaspoon vegetable oil
- ½ tablespoon minced garlic
- ¼ cup water
- ¼ teaspoon ground ginger
- ¼ cup soy sauce
- 6 tablespoons packed brown sugar

<u>To serve:</u>

- Cooked or air fried green beans
- 1 green onion, thinly sliced
- Hot rice

Method:

1. Spread cornstarch on a plate. Dredge the steak slices in cornstarch. Shake to drop off excess cornstarch. Place in the air fryer basket.

2. Grill in a preheated air fryer at 390 º F or about 8-10 minutes. Flip sides and grill the other side for 8-10 minutes.

3. Meanwhile, add all the ingredients for sauce into a saucepan. Place saucepan over medium heat. Whisk well. Turn off the heat when it begins to boil.

4. Remove the steak from the air fryer and place in a bowl. Pour the sauce over the steak. Turn the steak and let it rest for a few minutes.

5. To serve: Place cooked rice on a serving platter. Place steak over the rice (shake off the sauce if desired). Serve with green beans.

Teriyaki Steak with Hassel back Potatoes

Serves: 1

Ingredients:

- 2 medium sized potatoes, peeled, cut a thin slice so that it can stand
- 1 steak, cut into strips
- ½ cup snow peas
- 1 medium onion, halved, sliced
- 1 teaspoon soy sauce
- Salt or to taste
- Pepper to taste
- 5 ounces mushrooms, quartered
- 2 tablespoons olive oil
- 2 teaspoons ketjap manis sauce (a thick, sweet, Indonesian soy sauce)

Method:

1. Make small slits on the potatoes with a sharp knife. Drizzle some oil in the slits. Season the potatoes with salt and pepper.
2. Place the potatoes in the baking accessory.

3. Place the baking accessory in the air fryer.
4. Roast in a preheated air fryer at 390 º F or about 20 minutes.
5. Meanwhile, mix together rest of the ingredients and marinate for a while.
6. Push the potatoes to one side and place the marinated ingredients in the middle.
7. Roast for 5 more minutes.
8. Serve potatoes with the vegetable - steak mixture.

Cheesy Lasagna

Serves: 2

Ingredients:

For meat layer:

- ½ pound 85% lean ground beef
- 2 tablespoons chopped celery
- 1 clove garlic, minced
- Extra-virgin olive oil, as required
- ½ cup marinara sauce
- 2 tablespoons chopped onion
- Salt to taste
- Pepper to taste

For cheese layer:

- 4 ounces ricotta cheese
- ¼ cup grated Parmesan cheese
- ½ teaspoon dried Italian seasoning
- ½ cup shredded mozzarella cheese, divided
- 1 large egg
- 1 clove garlic, minced

Method:

1. To make meat layer: Grease the baking accessory or a baking dish with a little olive oil.
2. Add all the ingredients for meat layer into a bowl and mix until well incorporated.
3. Transfer into the prepared dish.
4. Place the dish tin the air fryer basket.
5. Bake in a preheated air fryer at 375 º F or about 10 minutes.
6. To make cheese layer: Add ricotta, Parmesan, ¼ cup mozzarella, seasoning, egg and garlic into a bowl and mix well.
7. Spread it evenly on top of the meat layer. Scatter the remaining mozzarella cheese.
8. Bake for another 8-10 minutes or until the internal temperature of meat shows 160 º F.
9. Discard the fat remaining in the baking dish. Let it rest for 5 minutes.
10. Serve.

Stuffed Cheeseburgers

Serves: 4

Ingredients:

- 1 ½ pounds lean ground beef
- 8 teaspoons ketchup

- Freshly ground pepper to taste
- Salt to taste
- 1/3 cup onions, minced
- 8 slices cheddar cheese, chopped
- 4 teaspoons yellow mustard
- 16 hamburger dill pickle chips

To serve:

- 4 hamburger buns, split
- Lettuce leaves
- Tomato slices
- Mayonnaise etc.

Method:

1. Add beef, onions, mustard, salt, pepper and ketchup into a bowl and mix well. Divide the mixture into 8 equal portions and shape into balls.
2. Take one portion and flatten it. Place 4 pickle chips on it. Place some cheese cubes. Take another portion, flatten it and cover the cheese. Press firmly on the edges.
3. Repeat the previous step and make the remaining 3 burgers.
4. Place the burgers in the air fryer basket.
5. Grill in a preheated air 370° F for 20 minutes. Flip the burgers half way through cooking.
6. Spread mayonnaise over the cut part of the buns.
7. Serve the burgers over buns with lettuce leaves and tomato slices.

Beef Empanadas

Serves: 2

Ingredients:

- ½ pound ground beef
- ½ tablespoon olive oil
- ½ small onion, minced
- 2 tablespoons chopped green bell pepper
- 1 clove garlic, peeled, minced
- 2-3 tablespoons tomato salsa
- 1 tablespoon milk
- Yolk of an egg
- ½ package empanada dough or also called shells
- ¼ teaspoon ground cumin
- Salt to taste
- Pepper to taste

Method:

1. Place a pan over high heat. Add oil and heat. Add beef and sauté until brown. Discard any extra fat that is remaining in the pan.
2. Add onion and garlic and stir. Cover and cook for 2-3 minutes.
3. Add salt, pepper, green bell pepper, salsa and cumin and mix well.

4. Lower the heat and cook for 7-8 minutes.

5. Add egg and milk into a bowl. Whisk well.

6. Place the empanada dough on your countertop. Roll with a rolling pin into small circles of 5-6 cm diameter.

7. Place about 1-½ tablespoons of the meat mixture on one half of the rolled dough. Brush the edges with the egg mixture. Fold the other half over the meat and press the edges to seal.

8. Now brush the empanada all over with the egg mixture.

9. Repeat steps 6-8 and fill the remaining shells.

10. Roast in a preheated air fryer at 350 $^\circ$ F or about 10 minutes or until crisp and brown.

11. Serve.

Steak Sandwiches

Serves: 2

Ingredients:

- 6 ounces top sirloin steak
- Salt to taste
- Pepper to taste
- ½ tablespoon garlic, minced
- 2 ½ tablespoons olive oil, divided
- 2 French rolls
- ¼ cup mayonnaise
- 1 tablespoon chopped parsley

Method:

1. Brush steak with 1 ½ tablespoons oil. Rub it well into it.
2. Sprinkle with salt and pepper all over the steak and place in the air fryer basket.
3. Grill in a preheated air fryer at 325 º F for about 10-12 minutes. Flip sides half way through grilling.
4. Remove the steaks and place on your cutting board. When cool enough to handle, slice the steak.
5. Place French rolls in the air fryer. Toast for 3-5 minutes depending on the desired doneness.

6. Meanwhile, add remaining oil, mayonnaise, parsley, garlic, salt and pepper into a blender and blend until it is emulsified.
7. Transfer into a bowl.
8. Remove steak from the air fryer and place on your cutting board. Slice the steak.
9. Spread the mayonnaise mixture over the French rolls. Place the steak over it and serve.
10. Serve with air baked onions and peppers.

Thai Beef Salad

Serves: 2

Ingredients:

<u>For salad:</u>

- 2 Porterhouse steaks
- 1 small cucumber, thinly sliced
- 3 1/2 ounces cherry tomatoes, quartered
- 1 small spring onion, thinly sliced
- ½ cup fresh mint leaves
- ½ cup fresh Thai basil
- 1 long fresh red chili, deseeded, thinly sliced
- ½ cup chopped cilantro
- Roasted peanuts, chopped, to serve

<u>For dressing:</u>

- Juice of a lime
- ½ tablespoon brown sugar
- 1 teaspoon sesame oil
- 1 teaspoon finely grated ginger
- ½ tablespoon fish sauce
- 1 tablespoon soy sauce
- 1 clove garlic, crushed

Method:

1. Add all the ingredients for dressing into a bowl and whisk until well combined. Cover and set aside for a while for the flavors to set in.
2. Pour half the dressing into a bowl and set aside.
3. Place steak in the remaining dressing. Let it marinate for 2-5 hours.
4. Remove steak from the marinade and sprinkle salt and pepper over it.
5. Place steak in the air fryer basket.
6. Grill in a preheated air fryer at 325° F for about 8-10, depending on the desired doneness. Flip sides half way through grilling.
7. Remove the steaks and place on your cutting board. When cool enough to handle, thinly slice the steak.
8. Add rest of the salad ingredients into a bowl and toss well.
9. Place steak over the salad. Drizzle any of the cooked juices over the salad. Also drizzle the retained dressing over the salad.
10. Serve.

Chapter Three: Air Fryer Fish Recipes

Hot Smoked Trout Frittata

Serves: 2

Ingredients:

- 1 onion, sliced
- 1 tablespoon olive oil
- 3 eggs
- 1 teaspoon horseradish sauce
- 1 tablespoon crème fraiche
- 1 hot smoked trout fillet
- Salt to taste
- Pepper to taste
- 2 tablespoons chopped fresh dill

Method:

1. Place a skillet over medium heat. Add oil and heat. Add onions and sauté until translucent. Transfer into the baking accessory or a small baking dish that can fit well into the air fryer.
2. Place the trout over the onion.

3. Whisk the eggs in a bowl. Add crème fraiche and horseradish and whisk well. Pour over the trout and onions. Sprinkle salt and pepper over it.

4. Air fry in a preheated air fryer at 320° F for 20 minutes or until set.

5. Sprinkle dill on top. Cut into wedges and serve.

Grilled Salmon Steaks

Serves: 2

Ingredients:

- 1 clove garlic, chopped
- A handful fresh cilantro, chopped
- 1 spring onion, thinly sliced
- 1 tablespoon French mustard
- 2 salmon steaks
- Juice of ½ lime
- 2 small tomatoes, chopped
- 2 tablespoons honey
- Salt to taste
- Pepper to taste

Method:

1. Add tomatoes, a little cilantro and spring onions into a bowl.
2. Add honey, lime juice, garlic, mustard, salt, pepper and a little cilantro into a small pan. Place pan over low heat. Stir frequently until the honey is well blended into the mixture. Turn off the heat and let it cool for a while.
3. Place salmon steaks in a shallow bowl. Pour the honey mixture over the salmon.
4. Turn the salmon and coat the other side too.

5. Remove salmon steaks from the marinade and shake to drop off excess marinade.
6. Grill in a preheated air fryer at 325 º F for about 7-10, depending on the desired doneness. Flip sides half way through grilling.
7. Place salmon on serving plates. Divide the tomato salad over the salmon.
8. Serve with hot rice and snow peas.

Cajun Salmon

Serves: 2

Ingredients:

- 2 fresh salmon fillets
- ½ teaspoon sugar (optional)
- Cajun seasoning, as required
- Lemon juice to taste

Method:

1. Place Cajun seasoning in a plate. Spread it all over. Sprinkle sugar if using. Dredge the fillet on both the sides. Place in the grill, with the skin side facing up.
2. Grill in a preheated air fryer at 350 º F for about 7-10, depending on the desired doneness.
3. Drizzle lemon juice on top and serve.

Baked Butter Crayfish

Serves: 6

Ingredients:

- 6 crayfish, rinsed, scrubbed
- 6 small cubes butter
- 6 small cream cubes
- 2 teaspoons garlic powder
- ¼ teaspoon salt or to taste
- ¼ teaspoon pepper powder
- Cooked spaghetti with sauce of your choice, to serve (optional)

Method:

1. Place a sheet of aluminum foil on your countertop. Place the crayfish with its bottom side up.
2. Place butter and cream cubes all over the crayfish.
3. Season with salt, pepper and garlic powder.
4. Wrap the crayfish with sides of the foil. It should be well sealed.
5. Place the sealed crayfish packet in the air fryer basket.
6. Air fry in a preheated air fryer at 375° F for 18 to 20 minutes.
7. Serve with spaghetti and a spaghetti sauce of your choice if desired.

Salmon Cakes

Serves: 4

Ingredients:

- 4 cans (7.5 ounces each) unsalted pink salmon with skin and bones, drained
- ¼ cup chopped, fresh dill
- 4 teaspoons Dijon mustard
- 2 large eggs
- 1 cup whole wheat panko breadcrumbs
- 4 tablespoons mayonnaise
- Pepper to taste
- Lemon wedges to serve

Method:

1. Remove any large bones and skin from the salmon and add into a bowl. Add rest of the ingredients and mix until well incorporated.
2. Divide the mixture into 4 equal portions and shape into patties.
3. Spray the cakes on both the sides with cooking spray and place in the air fryer basket.
4. Grill in a preheated air fryer at 350 º F for about 7-12, depending on the desired doneness.
5. Flip sides half way through grilling.

6. Serve with a dip of your choice.

Crumbed Fish

Serves: 2

Ingredients:

- 2 flounder fish fillets
- 2 tablespoons vegetable oil
- Salt to taste (optional)
- Pepper to taste (optional)
- 1 small egg, beaten
- ½ cup dry breadcrumbs
- Lemon wedges to serve

Method:

1. Add breadcrumbs, oil, salt, and pepper in a bowl. Mix until crumbly.
2. First dip the fish in egg. Shake to drop off the excess egg. Next dredge the fillets in the breadcrumbs mixture and place in the air fryer basket.
3. Air fry in a preheated air fryer at 370° F for 12 minutes or until the desired doneness.
4. Serve with lemon wedges.

Grilled Fish with Light Mayo Sauce

Serves: 2

Ingredients:

- 2 fish fillets
- ½ teaspoon smoked paprika
- ½ teaspoon ground coriander
- 1 tablespoon vegetable oil
- ½ red bell pepper, deseeded
- Lemon juice to taste
- 2 tablespoon light mayonnaise
- ½ tablespoon olive oil
- Salt to taste
- Pepper to taste
- ½ teaspoon ground cumin
- ¼ teaspoon ground ginger
- 2 tablespoons chopped fresh cilantro

Method:

1. Brush bell pepper with oil and place in the air fryer basket.
2. Grill in a preheated air fryer at 350 ° F for about 12-15 minutes, until slightly charred.
3. Remove the pepper from the air fryer and place in a bowl. Cover the bowl with plastic wrap and let it rest for 10-12

minutes. Remove the pepper and peel off the skin. Place on your cutting board and chop into fine pieces.

4. Transfer into a bowl. Also add olive oil, mayonnaise, salt, pepper, cilantro and a little lemon juice into a bowl. Mix well. Cover and set aside for a while for the flavors to set in.

5. Add vegetable oil, coriander, cumin, lemon juice, pepper, paprika and salt into a bowl and stir well. Rub this mixture onto the fish fillets and place in the air fryer.

6. Grill in a preheated air fryer at 350 º F for about 12-15 minutes, depending on the desired doneness.

7. Flip sides half way through grilling.

8. Serve with chilled mayonnaise sauce mixture.

Teriyaki Glazed Halibut Steak

Serves: 1-2

Ingredients:

- ½ pound halibut steak

For the marinade:

- 1/3 cup low sodium soy sauce
- 2 tablespoons sugar
- 2 tablespoons orange juice
- 4 tablespoons mirin, (Japanese cooking wine)
- 1 tablespoon lime juice
- 1/8 teaspoon ground ginger
- 1/8 teaspoon chili flakes, crushed
- 1 garlic clove, smashed

Method:

1. Place a saucepan over medium heat. Add all the ingredients of the marinade into the saucepan and bring to a boil.
2. Boil until the marinade is reduced to half its original quantity. Turn off the heat and set aside to cool.
3. Place the halibut in a Ziploc bag.
4. Slowly pour marinade over the halibut. Seal the bag and shake to coat well.

5. Chill for about 30-40 minutes.

6. Place the halibut in the air fryer basket.

7. Air fry in a preheated air fryer at 390° F for 10- 12 minutes.

8. Place steak over rice.

9. Pour the remaining glaze over the halibut and serve hot with basil or mint chutney if desired.

Salmon Quiche

Serves: 4

Ingredients:

- 10-11 ounces salmon fillet, cubed
- Freshly ground pepper to taste
- 3 1/2 ounces cold butter, cubed
- 6 tablespoons whipping cream
- 7 ounces flour
- 4 eggs
- 2 yolks
- 2 tablespoons mustard
- 1 tablespoon lemon juice
- 2 green onions, sliced into ½ inch pieces
- Salt to taste

Method:

1. Add salmon, salt, pepper and lemon juice into a bowl and mix well. Set aside for a while to marinate.
2. Add flour, yolks, about 2 tablespoons water and butter into a mixing bowl and knead into smooth dough.
3. Divide the dough into 2 equal portions and shape into balls.

4. Dust your countertop with a little flour. Roll the dough on your countertop to about 7-8 inches diameter.

5. Take 2 quiche pans that can fit well inside the air fryer and place rolled dough in each. Press it well onto the bottom as well as sides of the pan.

6. Add eggs, mustard, cream, salt, and pepper into a bowl and beat lightly until well incorporated. Pour into the quiche pans. Place the salmon cubes all over the quiche. Sprinkle green onion all over, as well. Bake in batches.

7. Bake in a preheated air fryer at 350° F for 20 minutes or until golden brown.

8. Cut into wedges and serve.

Southern Style Catfish with Green Beans

Serves: 1

Ingredients:

- 6 ounces fresh green beans, trimmed
- ½ teaspoon light brown sugar
- Salt to taste
- 2 tablespoons all-purpose flour
- 3 tablespoons panko bread crumbs
- 1 tablespoon mayonnaise
- ½ teaspoon dill pickle relish
- A pinch granulated sugar
- ¼ teaspoon crushed red pepper (optional)
- 1 catfish fillet
- 1 small egg, lightly beaten
- Pepper to taste
- 1 teaspoon minced fresh dill
- ¼ teaspoon apple cider vinegar
- Lemon wedges to serve

Method:

1. Add green beans, brown sugar, salt and crushed red pepper into a bowl. Toss well.

2. Spray some cooking spray generously over the beans and toss well.

3. Transfer into the air fryer basket.

4. Roast in a preheated air fryer at 400° F for 12 minutes or until brown and tender as well.

5. Remove from the air fryer and place in a bowl. Cover the bowl with foil and set aside.

6. Dredge catfish in flour. Shake to drop off excess flour. Next dip in egg. Shake to drop off excess egg. Finally dredge in panko breadcrumbs and place in the air fryer basket.

7. Spray the fillet with some cooking spray.

8. Roast in a preheated air fryer at 400° F for 8 minutes or until cooked through inside and crisp outside.

9. Remove from the air fryer and season with salt.

10. Meanwhile, add mayonnaise, vinegar, sugar, dill and dill pickle relish in a bowl and whisk until sugar dissolves completely.

11. Serve roasted catfish fillet with roasted green beans, lemon wedges and sauce.

Fish en Papillotte

Serves: 4

Ingredients:

- 4-5 fingerling potatoes, sliced into ¼ inch thick slices

- ¼ cup butter, melted
- 1 cup julienned bulb fennel
- 1 cup julienned carrot
- 1 cup thinly sliced red bell pepper
- Freshly ground pepper to taste
- Salt to taste
- 4 cod fillets (5 ounces each)
- 2 tablespoons lemon juice
- 2 tablespoons oil

Method:

1. Add butter, tarragon, salt and lemon juice into a bowl and stir. Add vegetables and stir.
2. Place 4 large squares of parchment paper on your countertop.
3. Spray the fillets with oil. Season with salt and pepper and place a fillet on each sheet of parchment paper. Divide and place the vegetables over the fillets.
4. Fold the parchment paper over the fillets to make into packets.
5. Place the packets in the air fryer in batches.
6. Air fry in a preheated air fryer at 350° F for about 15 minutes. Remove from the air fryer and let it rest for 3-4 minutes.
7. Open the packets and serve.

Grilled Fish Fillets with Pesto Sauce

Serves: 6

Ingredients:

- ¼ cup pine nuts
- 6 white fish fillets
- Salt to taste
- Pepper to taste
- 4 cloves garlic
- 2 tablespoons grated Parmesan cheese
- 2 tablespoons olive oil
- 2 bunches fresh basil, chopped
- 1 cup extra virgin olive oil

Method:

1. Brush olive oil over the fish fillets. Sprinkle salt and pepper over the fillets.
2. Place the fish fillets in the air fryer basket.
3. Grill in a preheated air fryer at 350° F for 8 minutes.
4. To make pesto sauce: Blend together basil, garlic, pine nuts, extra-virgin olive oil, Parmesan cheese, salt, pepper and olive oil until smooth.
5. Serve the fillets with pesto sauce.

Broiled Tilapia

Serves: 4

Ingredients:

- 2 pounds tilapia fillets, thaw if frozen
- 1 teaspoon old bay seasoning or to taste
- A pinch salt or to taste
- 1 teaspoon lemon pepper
- ¼ teaspoon smoked paprika
- ½ tablespoon olive oil
- Butter buds, as required

Method:

1. Drizzle oil over the fillets. Sprinkle all the spices over the fillets. Rub it well into the fillets.
2. Place fillets in the air fryer basket. Spray some cooking spray over the fillets.
3. Airy fry in a preheated air fryer at 350° F for 7-8 minutes.
4. Serve with vegetables of your choice.

Roasted Salmon with Fennel Salad

Serves: 2

Ingredients:

- 1 teaspoon finely chopped fresh flat-leaf parsley
- ½ teaspoon kosher salt, divided
- 1 tablespoon olive oil
- 1/3 cup low fat, 2% Greek yogurt
- 1 tablespoon fresh orange juice
- 1 tablespoon chopped fresh dill
- ½ teaspoon minced fresh thyme
- 2 salmon fillets, skinless, center-cut
- 2 cups thinly sliced fennel
- 1 small clove garlic, peeled, grated
- ½ teaspoon fresh lemon juice

Method:

1. Add salt and herbs in a bowl and mix well.
2. Brush oil over the salmon. Scatter the herb mixture over it and place in the air fryer basket.
3. Airy fry in a preheated air fryer at 350° F for 8-10 minutes depending on you like it cooked.
4. Meanwhile, add rest of the ingredients into a bowl and stir until well combined.

5. Divide fennel salad into 2 plates. Place salmon fillets on top and serve.

Thai Fish Cakes with Mango Salsa

Serves: 2-3

Ingredients:

For fish cake:

- 9 ounces fish fillets
- 1 small egg
- ½ teaspoon red chili paste
- 2 tablespoon finely chopped green onion
- 2 tablespoons ground coconut + extra to dredge
- Juice of ½ lime
- ¼ teaspoon grated lime zest
- A handful fresh flat leaf parsley or cilantro, chopped
- Salt to taste

For mango salsa:

- 2 medium ripe mangoes, peeled, cut into small cubes
- ¼ teaspoon red chili paste
- Salt to taste
- Juice of ½ lime
- ¼ teaspoon grated zest lime
- A handful fresh flat leaf parsley or cilantro, chopped

Method:

1. To make the mango salsa: Mix together in a bowl, mango, 1 teaspoon chili paste, a little cilantro leaves, remaining lime juice, and lime zest. Mix well and set aside for a while for the flavors to set in.

2. To make fish cakes: Add fish, lime zest, egg, salt, red chili paste, coconut and lime juice into the food processor bowl and pulse until well combined.

3. Transfer into a bowl. Add cilantro and green onion. Divide the mixture into 2-3 equal portions and shape into patties.

4. Place fish cakes in the air fryer basket. Place the basket in the air fryer.

5. Airy fry in a preheated air fryer at 350° F for 7-8 minutes depending on you like it cooked.

6. Serve fish cakes with mango salsa.

Crispy Cod Nuggets

Serves: 4-8

Ingredients:

- 2 pounds cod fillets, cut into chunks
- 1 cup flour
- 2 cups cracker fine crumbs or finely crushed cornflakes
- Salt to taste

- Pepper to taste
- 1 egg whisked with 2 tablespoons water
- 2 tablespoon vegetable oil

For lemon honey tartar sauce:

- 1 cup low fat mayonnaise
- 2 tablespoons dill pickle relish
- 2 teaspoons honey
- ¼ teaspoon crushed red pepper (optional)
- Juice of ½ lemon
- ¼ teaspoon grated lemon zest
- ¼ teaspoon Worcestershire sauce
- Pepper to taste

Method:

1. You can crush the crackers or cornflakes in the food processor.
2. Place cod chunks in a bowl. Sprinkle salt and pepper over it. Toss well.
3. Place flour in a shallow bowl. Add cod chunks and coat it well in the mixture. Shake to drop off excess flour.
4. Now dip the chunks in the egg mixture. Shake to drop off excess egg.
5. Finally dredge in the cracker crumbs.
6. Place in the air fryer basket.
7. Airy fry in a preheated air fryer at 350° F for 15 minutes or until crisp.
8. Meanwhile, add all the ingredients for honey tartar sauce into a bowl and whisk well. Set aside for a while for the flavors to set in.
9. Serve with air fried French fries and honey tartar sauce.

Salmon Patties

Serves: 10-12

Ingredients:

- 1.8 pounds russet potatoes, peeled, chopped into small pieces
- 1 cup frozen vegetables, parboiled, drained
- 1 pound salmon
- 2 teaspoons dried dill
- Salt to taste
- Pepper to taste
- 2 eggs
- 2 tablespoons chopped fresh parsley
- Bread crumbs as required
- Mayonnaise to serve
- Lemon wedges to serve

Method:

1. Place a pot of water over medium heat. Add potatoes and bring to a boil. Simmer until potatoes are tender.
2. Drain the water and add the potatoes back into the pot. Place the pot over low heat until dry. Remove from heat and transfer into a large mixing bowl. Mash with a potato masher. Chill for 15 minutes.
3. Meanwhile, place the salmon in the air fryer basket.

4. Grill in a preheated air fryer at 350° F for 5 minutes or until brown. Remove from the air fryer and cool slightly. When cool enough to handle, flake the salmon with a fork and set aside.

5. Remove the potatoes from the refrigerator and add vegetables, salmon, parsley, dill, salt and pepper. Mix until well combined. Taste and adjust the seasoning if necessary.

6. Add eggs and mix well. Divide the mixture into 10 to 12 equal portions and shape into patties.

7. Line the air fryer basket with aluminum foil or you can use a grill pan.

8. Dredge the patties in breadcrumbs and place in the air fryer basket. Spray with cooking spray.

9. Grill in a preheated air fryer at 350° F for 12 minutes or until brown. Flip sides half way through cooking.

10. Serve with mayonnaise, lemon wedges with a salad of your choice.

Easy Salmon Fried Rice

Serves: 2

Ingredients:

- 2 rice bowls cooked rice (a day old)
- 2-3 ounces crab meat
- 1 salmon fillet (3-4 ounces)
- A handful shredded cabbage
- 1 carrot, cut into thin strips
- ½ cup frozen corn, thawed, blanched, drained
- 1 shallot, minced
- 1 egg, whisked
- ½ tablespoon minced garlic
- ½ teaspoon soy sauce
- 1 tablespoon oyster sauce
- ½ teaspoon fish sauce
- 1 tablespoon olive oil
- ½ teaspoon sugar

Method:

1. Place the fillet in the air fryer basket.
2. Airy fry in a preheated air fryer at 370 º F for 7 minutes.
3. Remove the fillet and place on your cutting board. Flake the fillet with a fork.

4. Place a wok over high heat. Add oil and heat. Add shallot and sauté until translucent. Add garlic and sauté for a few seconds until aromatic.

5. Add carrots and cabbage and sauté for 3 minutes.

6. Add crabmeat and corn. Stir-fry for a couple of minutes.

7. Add rice, sugar, soy sauce, oyster sauce and fish sauce and toss until well combined.

8. Push the mixture to the sides of the wok making space in the center. Add egg in the center. Do not stir for 20 seconds.

9. Push the rice mixture back to the center. Stir the entire ingredients in the wok until the eggs are well distributed.

10. Add salmon and mix well.

11. Serve.

Black Cod with Grapes, Fennel, Pecans and Kale

Serves: 4

Ingredients:

- 4 (6 to 8 ounces each) black cod fillets
- 2 small bulb fennels, sliced into ¼ inch thick slices
- 6 cups kale, discard hard stems and ribs, shredded
- 4 tablespoons extra- virgin olive oil
- Freshly ground pepper to taste
- Salt to taste
- 2 cups grapes, halved
- 1 cup pecans
- 4 teaspoons white wine vinegar or balsamic vinegar

Method:

1. Sprinkle salt and pepper over the fillets. Spray cooking spray over the fillets.
2. Place the fillets in the air fryer basket.
3. Air fry in a preheated air fryer at 390° F for 10 minutes.
4. Brush with oil and fry for another 5 minutes.
5. Remove from the air fryer and place on a plate. Cover loosely with foil and set aside for a while.
6. Mix together in a bowl, grapes, pecans, salt, pepper and fennel. Pour about a tablespoon olive oil over it. Toss well.

7. Transfer into the air fryer basket.

8. Air fry in a preheated air fryer at 390° F for 5 minutes. Shake the basket half way through cooking.

9. Transfer into a bowl. Add kale and toss.

10. Whisk together in a bowl, vinegar, 3 tablespoons olive oil, salt and pepper. Pour over kale. Toss well.

11. Serve fish with the grape salad.

Lemon Fish

Serves: 2

Ingredients:

- 1 basa fish fillet, quartered
- ½ cup all-purpose flour + extra for dredging
- Juice of ½ lemon
- 1 lemon, cut into slices
- 1 teaspoon green chili sauce
- 1 teaspoon red chili sauce
- 1 small egg white
- 2 tablespoons sugar
- 1 cup water
- 2 teaspoons cornstarch mixed with 1 tablespoon water
- 1 teaspoon oil + extra for brushing
- Salt to taste
- Few lettuce leaves, torn

Method:

1. Add sugar and water into a pan. Place the pan over medium heat. Bring to the boil. Stir until the sugar dissolves.

2. Add salt, red chili sauce, lemon juice, and lemon slices. Stir well. Add cornstarch mixture and stir constantly until the mixture thickness. Turn off the heat.

3. Meanwhile, brush fish fillets with a little oil. Sprinkle salt and pepper over it.

4. Add flour, salt, green chili sauce, oil, egg white, and 1 ½ tablespoons water into a bowl and whisk until smooth batter is formed. Set aside.

5. Place flour in a bowl. First dip the fish in the batter. Shake the fish to drop off excess batter. Next dredge in flour. Shake again to drop off excess flour and place in the air fryer basket.

6. Air fry in a preheated air fryer at 390° F for 15-20 minutes.

7. Brush again some oil over the fish and fry for another 5 minutes.

8. To serve: Place fried fish over a bed of lettuce leaves. Pour lemon sauce over it and serve.

Fish Taco

Serves: 3

Ingredients:

<u>For the fish tacos:</u>

- 5 ounces cod fillets, cut into 3 long pieces
- White pepper powder to taste
- ½ cup coleslaw
- ¼ cup guacamole
- Lemon wedges to serve
- ½ cup panko bread crumbs
- 3 large tortillas
- 2 tablespoons cheese, shredded (optional)
- ¼ cup salsa
- Salt to taste
- A handful fresh cilantro, chopped

<u>To make tempura batter:</u>

- ½ cup flour
- ¼ teaspoon salt or to taste
- ¾ cup water
- ½ tablespoon cornstarch

Method:

1. To make tempura batter: Add all the ingredients of tempura batter into a bowl and whisk well.

2. Cut the fillets into 2 ounce long pieces. Sprinkle salt and pepper to taste.

3. First dip the fish pieces in tempura batter. Shake to drop off excess batter. Next dredge in panko breadcrumbs. Shake to drop off excess breadcrumbs.

4. Place the fish pieces in the air fryer basket.

5. Air fry in a preheated air fryer at 390° F for 6-7 minutes.

6. To assemble: Place the tortillas on your countertop. Smear guacamole over the tortillas.

7. Place a fish piece on each tortilla and top with salsa, coleslaw, fresh cilantro and some lemon juice.

8. Wrap the tortillas and serve.

9. If you want crispy tortillas, then place the rolled tortillas with the seam side down in the air fryer basket and fry for a few minutes until crisp.

10. Serve with some more guacamole or salsa.

Salmon with Creamy Courgetti

Serves: 4

Ingredients:

- 4 salmon fillets (6 ounces each) with skin
- 4 teaspoons oil
- 2 ripe avocadoes, peeled, pitted, chopped
- 2-3 tablespoons parsley, chopped
- 2 handfuls black olives, sliced
- 4 large, straight courgettes, trimmed
- 1 clove garlic, finely chopped
- 2 handfuls cherry tomatoes, chopped
- 4 tablespoons pine nuts, toasted
- Salt to taste
- Pepper to taste

Method:

1. Rub oil over the salmon fillets. Sprinkle salt and pepper over it.
2. Place the fillet in the air fryer basket.
3. Air fry in a preheated air fryer at 390° F for 6-7 minutes.
4. Meanwhile, make noodles of the courgette with a spiralizer or a julienne peeler.
5. Add avocado, parsley, garlic, salt and pepper into a blender and blend until smooth.

6. Transfer into a bowl. Add courgette and toss until well coated.

7. Serve creamy courgette with tomatoes and salmon. Sprinkle pine nuts on top and serve.

Fish Finger Sandwich

Serves: 2

Ingredients:

- 2 small cod fillets, skinless
- 1 tablespoon flour
- 4 1/2 ounces frozen peas
- 5-6 capers
- 2 bread rolls or 4 small bread slices
- Salt to taste
- Pepper to taste
- Breadcrumbs, as required
- ½ tablespoon crème fraiche or Greek yogurt
- Lemon juice to taste

To serve: Optional

- Lettuce
- Tomato slices
- Tartar sauce
- Any other toppings of your choice

Method:

1. Sprinkle salt and pepper over the fillets and lightly sprinkle flour over it.
2. Dredge in breadcrumbs, lightly. Shake to drop off excess breadcrumbs. Place in the air fryer basket.

3. Air fry in a preheated air fryer at 390° F for 15 minutes.

4. Meanwhile, place a small saucepan with water over medium heat. Add peas and cook until tender. Turn off the heat and drain off the water.

5. Add peas, crème fraiche, lemon juice and capers into a blender and blend until smooth.

6. If using rolls, split the rolls. Toast the rolls or bread slices if desired.

7. Spread pea mixture over the bread slices. Place a fillet each on 2 bread slices (or bottom half of rolls). Place the toppings you are using. Cover with remaining bread slices and serve.

Fish and Chips

Serves: 2

Ingredients:

- 1 large russet potato, scrubbed
- Salt to taste
- 1 large egg
- ½ cup whole wheat panko bread crumbs
- ¼ cup malt vinegar
- ½ cup all-purpose flour
- 1 tablespoon water
- 2 tilapia fillets (6 ounces each), skinless, halved lengthwise

Method:

1. Make spirals of the potatoes using a spiralizer.
2. Cook in batches. Spread potato spirals in the air fryer basket. Spray some cooking spray over it. Toss well and spray again until well coated.
3. Air fry in a preheated air fryer at 390° F for 10 minutes. Turn the potatoes halfway through frying.
4. Remove from the air fryer. Season with salt and set aside.
5. Meanwhile, add flour and a little salt in a shallow bowl.
6. Add eggs and water in another bowl and whisk well.
7. Add panko bread crumbs and salt in a third bowl
8. First roll the fish strips in flour mixture. Shake to drop off excess flour. Next dip in egg. Shake to drop off excess egg.

9. Finally roll in panko. Press it lightly so that the panko sticks onto the fish.

10. Spray the fish with cooking spray, all over and place in the air fryer basket.

11. Air fry in a preheated air fryer at 375° F for 10 minutes. Turn the fish halfway through frying.

12. Serve 2 slices of fish in each serving plate. Divide the potato spirals among the plates and serve with 2 tablespoons malt vinegar as a dip.

Mediterranean Fish Casserole

Serves: 2

Ingredients:

- 1 tablespoon olive oil
- 1 Italian frying peppers, thinly sliced
- Pepper to taste
- Salt to taste
- 2 cloves garlic, peeled, sliced
- 2 tablespoons pitted, chopped kalamata olives, chopped
- 1 tablespoon lemon juice
- 2 cod or halibut fillets (5-6 ounces each)
- ½ pound small white potatoes, quartered
- 1 plum tomato, deseeded, cut into ¼ inch wedges
- 2 tablespoons chopped, flat-leaf parsley

Method:

1. Grease the baking accessory or a small baking dish that can fit well inside the air fryer with cooking spray.
2. Scatter potatoes and Italian peppers all over the dish. Sprinkle salt and pepper.
3. Place the dish in the air fryer.
4. Roast in a preheated air fryer at 400° F for 30 minutes or until potatoes are tender. Turn the potatoes half way through baking.
5. Sprinkle garlic over the potatoes.

6. Sprinkle salt and pepper over the fish and place over the potatoes. Scatter the tomatoes and olives all over the baking dish. Sprinkle lemon juice and olive oil.

7. Bake for 20 minutes or until the fish is cooked through and flakes when pierced with a fork.

Chapter Four: Vegetarian Recipes

Mascarpone Mushroom Pasta

Serves: 2

Ingredients:

- 2 cups sliced mushrooms
- 1 teaspoon minced garlic
- 4 ounces mascarpone cheese, chopped
- ½ teaspoon pepper
- ¼ teaspoon red pepper flakes
- ½ cup chopped onion
- 2 tablespoons cream or half and half
- ½ teaspoon dried thyme
- ½ teaspoon salt
- ¼ cup shredded cheese
- 2 cups pasta

Method:

1. Grease the air fryer baking accessory or a small baking dish that can fit well into the air fryer with cooking spray.
2. Add mushrooms, garlic, mascarpone cheese, salt pepper, thyme, red pepper flakes, onion and cream into a bowl and stir. Transfer into the prepared baking dish.
3. Bake in a preheated air fryer at 350º F for 15 minutes. Stir once half way through baking.

4. Meanwhile, cook the pasta following the instructions on the package.
5. Place cooked pasta in a bowl. Top with mushroom mixture. Sprinkle cheese on top and serve.

Green Curry Noodles

Serves: 3

Ingredients:

- 1 pound shirataki noodles
- ¾ tablespoon fish sauce (optional)
- ¼ teaspoon garlic powder
- 2 1/2 ounces snow peas
- 10 ounces extra firm tofu, cubed
- 1 cup thinly sliced mushrooms
- 1 small green bell pepper, thinly sliced
- 1 small red bell pepper, thinly sliced
- ½ cup sliced water chestnuts
- 1 cup broccoli florets
- 6 ounces Napa cabbage
- 2 spring onions, thinly sliced
- 1 medium carrot, peeled, shredded
- ½ teaspoon ground coriander
- 1 teaspoon lemon grass paste
- 1 ½ tablespoons lemon juice
- 2 tablespoons rice vinegar
- 3 tablespoons Thai green curry paste or to taste
- ½ teaspoon sesame oil
- 3 tablespoons soy sauce

Method:

1. Drain the water from the shirataki noodles, if packed in water. Rinse with fresh running water. Transfer into a large bowl. Pour a cup of boiling water and 1-teaspoon soy sauce. Mix with a fork and set aside for a while.

2. To marinate tofu: Mix together in a bowl, half the soy sauce, and sesame oil and fish sauce and garlic powder. Add tofu and mix well.

3. To make the dressing: Add coriander, lime juice, 1 tablespoon rice vinegar, lemon grass paste and 2 tablespoons Thai curry paste into a bowl and mix well. Set aside.

4. Place a skillet over medium heat. Spray cooking spray over it. Add snow peas, peppers, water chestnuts, broccoli and mushrooms and sauté until tender. Remove from heat and set aside.

5. Mix together in a bowl, cabbage, carrots and spring onion. Set aside.

6. Remove the tofu from the marinade with a slotted spoon. Set aside the marinade and place tofu in the air fryer basket.

7. Spray tofu with cooking spray.

8. Air fry in a preheated air fryer at 360° F for about 12-13 minutes. Shake the basket a couple of times while frying. Transfer into a bowl and set aside.

9. To make stir fry sauce: Place a skillet or wok over medium heat. Add the retained tofu marinade, remaining vinegar and Thai curry paste. Stir until well combined.

Add the cabbage mixture and stir-fry for 2-3 minutes. Remove from heat.

10. Drain the noodles and place in a large bowl. Pour dressing on top. Add tofu and vegetables. Pour the stir-fry sauce over it. Toss using a pair of tongs.

11. Serve.

French Fries

Serves: 2

Ingredients:

- 2 large potatoes, peeled, chopped into fries
- 1 teaspoon oil
- Salt to taste
- Pepper to taste

Method:

1. Place the potatoes in a bowl of cold water for 30 minutes. Drain and dry the potatoes by patting with a kitchen towel.
2. Place the fries in a bowl and drizzle oil over it. Toss well.
3. Transfer into the air fryer basket.
4. Air fry in a preheated air fryer at 365° F for 25 minutes. Shake the basket a couple of times while frying.
5. Remove from the fryer and season with salt and pepper or any other seasoning of your choice and serve.

Italian Style Ratatouille

Serves: 2

Ingredients:

- ¼ yellow bell pepper, deseeded, chopped into ¾ inch squares
- ¼ red bell pepper, deseeded, chopped into ¾ inch squares
- 1 small tomato, deseeded chopped into ¾ inch cubes
- 1 zucchini, chopped into ¾ inch cubes
- 1 medium onion, chopped into ¾ inch cubes
- ¼ aubergine (eggplant), chopped into ¾ inch cubes
- ½ tablespoon olive oil
- 1 small clove garlic, crushed
- 1 small fresh cayenne pepper, chopped
- 1 sprig fresh oregano, chopped
- 3 sprigs fresh basil, chopped
- Freshly ground black pepper
- Salt to taste
- ½ teaspoon vinegar
- ½ tablespoon white wine

Method:

1. Mix together zucchini, aubergine, bell peppers, tomatoes, and onions in the air fryer baking accessory or a small baking dish that fits well into the air fryer.
2. Add garlic, oil, fresh cayenne pepper, vinegar, wine, herbs, salt and pepper. Mix well.
3. Place the baking dish in the air fryer basket.
4. Air fry in a preheated air fryer for 400° F 20-25 minutes or until tender. Stir the vegetables in between a couple of times. Remove from the air fryer and let it cool for 5 minutes.
5. Serve hot with air fried chicken or cutlets.

Roasted Vegetable Pasta Salad

Serves: 3-4

Ingredients:

- 1 medium eggplant, cut into ½ inch thick slices
- 1 medium zucchini, cut into ½ inch thick slices
- 1 medium tomato, cut into eighth
- 1 red or green bell pepper, chopped into 1 inch squares
- 1 ¼ cups dry large pasta
- 2 teaspoons olive oil
- ½ cup cherry tomatoes, halved
- 3 tablespoons Parmesan, grated
- Handful of basil, chopped
- ¼ cup low fat Italian dressing
- Salt to taste
- Pepper to taste

Method:

1. Drizzle a teaspoon of oil over the eggplant and place in the air fryer basket.
2. Roast in a preheated air fryer for 350° F for about 20-30 minutes or until soft.
3. Remove from the basket and set aside.
4. Toss zucchini with a teaspoon of oil and place in the air fryer basket.

5. Roast for about 20-30 minutes or until soft.
6. Remove from the basket and set aside.
7. Place tomatoes in the air fryer basket. Spray with cooking spray.
8. Roast for about 20-30 minutes or until it begins to brown.
9. Remove from the basket and set aside.
10. Meanwhile, cook the pasta following the instructions on the package. Transfer into a bowl.
11. Add all the ingredients into the bowl of pasta. Fold gently and chill for a couple of hours.
12. Stir and serve either chilled or at room temperature.

Green Beans with Spicy Dipping Sauce

Serves: 2

Ingredients:

For green beans:

- ½ cup all-purpose flour
- ½ cup beer
- 1 teaspoon salt
- 6 ounces fresh green beans, trimmed
- ¼ teaspoon pepper

For dipping sauce:

- ½ cup ranch dressing
- ½ teaspoon prepared horseradish or more to taste
- 1 teaspoon sriracha sauce

Method:

1. Add flour, beer, pepper and salt into a bowl and whisk until well combined.
2. Line the air fryer basket with parchment paper.
3. Dip green beans, a few at a time. Shake off excess batter and place in the air fryer basket. Cook in batches if required.

4. Air fry in a preheated air fryer for 400° F 8-10 minutes or until tender inside and crisp outside. Stir the beans a couple of times while frying.
5. To make dip: Add all the ingredients for dip into a bowl and whisk well.
6. Serve crispy green beans with dip.

Baked Potatoes

Serves: 4

Ingredients:

- 4 tablespoons peanut oil or butter, softened
- 4 large russet potatoes, scrubbed, rinsed,
- Coarse sea salt to taste
- Pepper to taste

Method:

1. Line the air fryer basket with aluminum foil.
2. Brush the potatoes with oil or butter and place in the air fryer basket. Sprinkle sea salt over the potatoes and place in the air fryer basket.
3. Bake in a preheated air fryer for 400° F 50-60 minutes or until tender inside. Turn the potatoes a couple of times while baking.
4. Brush the potatoes with a little butter or oil each time while turning the potatoes.
5. Serve hot seasoned with salt and pepper.

Spanakopita Bites

Serves: 4

Ingredients:

- 5 ounces baby spinach leaves
- 2 tablespoons 1% low-fat cottage cheese
- 1 tablespoon finely grated Parmesan cheese
- Zest of ½ lemon
- Pepper to taste
- A pinch cayenne pepper
- ½ tablespoon olive oil
- 1 tablespoon water
- 2 tablespoon crumbled feta cheese
- 1 small egg white
- ½ teaspoon dried oregano
- Kosher salt to taste
- 2 sheets frozen filo dough (13x18 inches), thawed

Method:

1. Place a pot of water over high heat. Bring to a boil. Add spinach and cook until it wilts. Drain and place in a colander. Squeeze the spinach of excess moisture and add into a bowl.
2. Add rest of the ingredients except oil and filo sheets into the bowl of spinach and mix well.

3. Place filo sheets on your countertop. Cut into each into 2 rectangles.

4. Brush oil on one piece. Place another filo piece over it. Brush again with oil. Repeat this until you have 4 layers of filo in all.

5. Now cut this filo layers into 4 strips, lengthwise of about 2 ¼ inches wide. Then cut each strip into 2 halves, crosswise. So now you have 8 strips in all.

6. Place a little of spinach mixture on one corner of the strip, in the shape of a triangle. Fold the corner with filling to form a triangle. Fold again into a triangle in a zigzag manner. Repeat making the triangle until the whole strip is used up. Apply water on the last edge and press well. Each strip will give you one triangle.

7. Repeat with the remaining strips. You get 8 filled triangles in all.

8. Spray the triangles with cooking spray. Place 4-5 triangles in the air fryer basket.

9. Bake in a preheated air fryer for 390° F 10-12 minutes or until golden brown.

10. Serve hot or warm or at room temperature.

Vegetable Spring Rolls

Serves: 5

Ingredients:

- 1 medium carrot, grated or thinly sliced
- 3 button mushrooms, thinly sliced
- ½ teaspoon minced ginger
- 1 small clove garlic, smashed
- ½ cup cabbage, thinly sliced
- 1/8 red bell pepper thinly sliced
- 1/8 yellow bell pepper thinly sliced
- 1 small green onion, thinly sliced
- ½ teaspoon soy sauce + extra to serve
- White pepper to taste
- 1 bird eye chili, thinly sliced
- ½ tablespoon vegetarian oyster sauce
- 5 spring roll wrappers
- 1 teaspoon vegetable oil + extra for brushing
- 2 tablespoons cornstarch mixed in 3 tablespoons water
- Sweet chili sauce to serve.

Method:

1. Place a nonstick skillet over medium heat. Add oil. When oil is heated, add green onions, ginger and garlic and sauté until aromatic.

167

2. Add carrots and sauté for a couple of minutes. Add cabbage and bell pepper and sauté for 2 minutes.

3. Add oyster sauce, pepper and soy sauce and stir-fry for a minute. Remove from heat. Add bird eye chili and stir. Let it cool a little.

4. Place the spring roll wrappers on your countertop. Divide and place the filling in the center of the wrappers. Spread it all along the center.

5. Apply cornstarch paste on the edges of the wrappers. Roll the wrappers and seal with the cornstarch paste. Press firmly to seal.

6. Brush the spring rolls with a little oil.

7. Place 2-3 spring rolls in the air fryer basket.

8. Air fry in a preheated air fryer at 390° F for 4 minutes or until golden brown.

9. Cook the remaining spring rolls in batches.

10. Serve with soy sauce and sweet chili sauce.

Crispy Vegetable Quesadilla

Serves: 2

Ingredients:

- 2 sprouted whole grain flour tortillas (6 inches each)
- ½ cup sliced, red bell pepper
- ½ cup unsalted canned or cooked black beans, drained, rinsed
- 1 ounce plain 2% reduced fat Greek yogurt
- 1/8 teaspoon ground cumin
- ¼ cup drained, refrigerated Pico de Gallo
- ½ cup shredded low fat sharp cheddar cheese
- ½ cup sliced zucchini
- ½ teaspoon grated lime zest
- ½ tablespoon fresh lime juice
- 1 tablespoon chopped, fresh cilantro

Method:

1. Spread the tortillas on your countertop. Scatter about 2 tablespoons of cheese on one half of each tortilla. Scatter zucchini, red pepper and black beans over the cheese. Sprinkle remaining cheese on top.
2. Fold the other half of the tortilla over the filling. Spray with cooking spray. Fasten with toothpicks.
3. Place in the air fryer basket.

169

4. Air fry in a preheated air fryer at 400° F for 10 minutes or until crisp. Flip sides half way through frying.

5. Meanwhile, make cumin cream as follows: Add yogurt, lime juice, lime zest and cumin into a bowl and whisk well.

6. Remove the quesadillas from the air fryer and cut into wedges. Garnish with cilantro and serve with cumin cream.

Beet Pumpkin and Goat Cheese Lasagna

Serves: 2

Ingredients:

- 12 1/3 ounces pumpkin, peeled, finely chopped
- 4 1/2 ounces mild goats cheese, grated (retain a little to garnish)
- 8 3/4 ounces beets, cooked, cut into thin slices (retain a couple of them to garnish)
- 14 ounces red tomatoes, chopped
- 3 tablespoons fresh rosemary, torn
- 4 1/2 ounces fresh lasagna sheets
- 1 tablespoon sunflower oil or olive oil
- ¼ cup grana padano cheese, grated
- 1 small onion, chopped

Method:

1. Place the pumpkin, onion and rosemary in a bowl and add about 2 tablespoons oil. Toss well and transfer it into the air fryer basket.
2. Roast in a preheated air fryer at 330° F for 10 minutes or until tender. Remove from the air fryer and cool slightly. Add the pumpkin mixture into a blender. Also add tomatoes and blend until smooth.

3. Pour the blended mixture into a pan. Place the pan over low heat and heat the sauce for 4-5 minutes.

4. Grease the baking accessory or a small baking dish that can fit well inside the air fryer with a little oil. Pour some of the sauce at the bottom of the dish. Place a layer of lasagna sheets on the bottom of the dish. Pour some more sauce over it. Layer with some beet slices followed by a sprinkle of goat's cheese.

5. Repeat the above layers (step 4) until all the ingredients are used up (retain some sauce and goats cheese for the topmost layer).

6. The top layers should be of sauce followed by goat's cheese.

7. Finally sprinkle grana padano cheese over the goat's cheese.

8. Bake in a preheated air fryer at 300° F for 45 minutes.

9. Garnish with some more goats' cheese and beet slices and serve.

Black Bean Burgers

Serves: 4-5

Ingredients:

- 1 can (15 ounces) black beans, drain off half the liquid
- 2 tablespoons chopped Roma tomatoes
- ½ teaspoon ground cumin
- ¼ cup breadcrumbs or panko breadcrumbs
- 1 small onion, minced
- Salt to taste
- Pepper to taste

Method:

1. Add beans into a bowl and mash with a fork.
2. Mix in rest of the ingredients until well combined. Mix with your hands.
3. Divide the mixture into 4-5 equal portions and shape into patties.
4. Place the burgers in the air fryer basket.
5. Grill in a preheated air fryer at 370° F for 8-10 minutes. Flip sides half way through grilling.
6. Serve with a dip of your choice.

Courgette Gratin

Serves: 2

Ingredients:

- 1 courgette, halved lengthwise first and then halved crosswise
- 1 tablespoon breadcrumbs
- 2 tablespoons grated cheese
- ½ tablespoon vegetable oil
- 1 tablespoon fresh parsley, chopped
- Pepper to taste
- Salt to taste

Method:

1. You are to get 4 pieces of courgette in all.
2. Mix together rest of the ingredients in a bowl. Place courgette pieces in the air fryer basket.
3. Divide and spread the cheese mixture over the courgette pieces.
4. Air fry in a preheated air fryer at 300° F for 15 minutes or until golden brown.

Potato Breakfast Gratin with Red Peppers & Parmesan

Serves: 3-4

Ingredients:

- 1 pound small red potatoes, cut into 1/8 to ¼ inch thick slices
- 2 cloves garlic, minced
- 5 large eggs
- ¼ cup yogurt
- Freshly ground pepper to taste
- Salt to taste
- 1 medium red bell pepper, finely chopped
- ¾ cup Parmesan cheese, divided
- ½ cup whole milk
- 2-3 tablespoons fresh parsley or basil to garnish

Method:

1. Grease the baking accessory or a baking dish that is smaller than the air fryer and fits well in the air fryer, with cooking spray.
2. Steam the potato slices until tender. Drain and place in the colander for a few minutes. You can also cook in a microwave.

3. Place half the slices in the prepared baking dish. Spread it evenly on the bottom of the dish, slightly overlapping if necessary.

4. Mix together in a bowl, bell pepper, half the cheese and garlic. Sprinkle over the potatoes.

5. Add eggs into a bowl and whisk well. Add yogurt, milk, remaining cheese, salt and pepper.

6. Pour half the egg mixture over the potatoes.

7. Place the remaining potatoes overlapping each other over the egg layer.

8. Pour remaining egg mixture on the potatoes.

9. Sprinkle remaining cheese on top.

10. Place the dish in the air fryer basket.

11. Bake in a preheated air fryer at 350° F for 15 minutes.

12. Let it rest in the air fryer for 8-10 minutes.

13. Sprinkle parsley and serve.

Roasted Rainbow Vegetables

Serves: 2

Ingredients:

- ½ red bell pepper, deseeded, cut into 1 inch squares
- 1 small zucchini, cut into 1 inch pieces
- 1 small sweet onion, cut into 1 inch thick wedges
- ½ yellow summer squash, cut into 1 inch pieces
- 2 ounces mushrooms, halved
- Salt to taste
- Pepper to taste
- ½ tablespoon extra-virgin olive oil

Method:

1. Toss together all the ingredients in a bowl.
2. Transfer into the air fryer basket.
3. Roast in a preheated air fryer at 330° F for 20-22 minutes or until tender. Turn the vegetables half way through roasting.
4. Serve hot or warm.

Eggplant Parmesan Sandwich

Serves: 1

Ingredients:

- 1 small eggplant (½ pound), cut into ½ inch slices
- ¼ cup bread crumbs
- ¼ teaspoon Italian seasoning
- ¼ teaspoon onion powder
- Freshly ground pepper, to taste
- ¼ cup mayonnaise
- 1 tablespoon milk
- 6 tablespoons tomato sauce
- 1 teaspoon dried parsley
- ¼ teaspoon garlic powder
- Salt to taste
- 1 tablespoon grated Parmesan cheese
- 1 cup grated mozzarella cheese
- 2 slices artisan Italian bread
- A handful fresh basil, chopped

Method:

1. Sprinkle salt generously over the eggplant slices and place it over paper towels. Set aside for 30 minutes.

2. Add breadcrumbs, seasoning, parsley, garlic powder, onion powder, pepper and salt into a shallow bowl and mix well.
3. Add milk and mayonnaise in another bowl. Whisk well.
4. Adjust the temperature of the air fryer to 390°F and preheat the air fryer.
5. Dip the eggplant slices in the mayonnaise mixture. Shake to drop off excess mixture. Next dredge in the breadcrumb mixture. Shake to drop off excess breadcrumbs.
6. Spray cooking spray on both the sides. Place in the air fryer basket. Cook in batches if required.
7. Air fry in a preheated air fryer at 400° F for 12-15 minutes. Flip sides half way through cooking. When done, remove from the basket.
8. Brush some oil generously on one side of bread slices Place some mozzarella cheese on one slice of bread, on the side that is not oiled. Place some Parmesan cheese, followed by eggplants. Spread some tomato sauce over it. Sprinkle remaining mozzarella cheese and Parmesan. Cover with the remaining slice with the oiled side facing up.
9. Fasten with toothpicks.
10. Grill in a preheated air fryer at 350° F for 15 minutes. Flip sides half way through grilling.

11. Cut each sandwich into 2 and serve with remaining tomato sauce.

Tofu Buddha Bowl

Serves: 3

Ingredients:

- 7 ounces extra-firm tofu
- 2 tablespoons soy sauce
- 1 tablespoon lime juice
- ½ pound fresh broccoli florets or Romanesco broccoli
- 1 small red bell pepper, thinly sliced
- 1 cup cooked red quinoa
- 1 tablespoon sesame oil
- 1 ½ tablespoons molasses or maple syrup
- ½ tablespoon sriracha sauce
- 3 small carrots, thinly sliced
- 4 ounces fresh spinach, stir-fried with olive oil and garlic
- Sesame seeds, to garnish

Method:

1. Place tofu over layers of paper towels. Cover with some layers of paper towels. Place something heavy on it like a heavy bottomed pan to drain out excess moisture. Let it sit in this position for 20-30 minutes.
2. Discard the paper towels and chop into very small cubes.
3. Mix together in a bowl, soy sauce, lime juice, sesame oil, molasses and sriracha sauce and whisk well.

4. Add tofu and mix well. Set aside for 10 minutes, to marinate. Stir once after 5 minutes.

5. Let the air fryer preheat for 3 minutes.

6. Remove tofu with a slotted spoon and place in the air fryer basket. Do not discard the marinade.

7. Air fry in a preheated air fryer at 370° F for 12-15 minutes. Shake the basket after every 5 minutes.

8. Add carrot, broccoli and bell pepper to the bowl of retained marinade. Mix well and let it marinate for 15 minutes.

9. Transfer tofu into a bowl. Remove vegetables with a slotted spoon and place in the air fryer basket. Do not discard the marinade.

10. Air fry for 10 minutes. Shake the basket after 5 minutes.

11. To serve: Divide quinoa among 3 serving bowls. Divide the vegetables equally and place over the quinoa.

12. Divide spinach and tofu among the bowls. Drizzle the retained marinade all over the bowls.

13. Sprinkle sesame seeds on top and serve.

Roasted Heritage Carrots and Rhubarb

Serves: 2

Ingredients:

- 1 teaspoon walnut oil
- ½ pound rhubarb
- ½ pound heritage carrots, chopped into chunks
- ¼ teaspoon stevia
- 1 small orange, separated into segments
- Zest of ½ orange, grated
- ¼ cup walnuts, chopped

Method:

1. Add carrots into the baking accessory or baking dish that is smaller than the air fryer and fits well in it. Sprinkle oil over it and toss.
2. Roast in a preheated air fryer at 350° F for 20 minutes.
3. Add rhubarb, stevia and walnuts and stir.
4. Roast for another for 6 minutes.
5. Add zest and oranges and stir.
6. Serve immediately.

Cauliflower Stir-Fry

Serves: 2

Ingredients:

- 1 small head cauliflower, cut into florets
- 3 cloves garlic, finely sliced
- ½ tablespoon rice vinegar
- ½ tablespoon sriracha or hot sauce of your choice
- 1 medium onion, thinly sliced
- ¾ tablespoon tamari
- ¼ teaspoon coconut sugar or sugar
- 1 scallion, sliced, to garnish

Method:

1. Place cauliflower in the baking accessory or baking dish that is smaller and that can fit well inside the air fryer.
2. Air fry in a preheated air fryer at 350° F for 10 minutes. Shake the basket after 5 minutes.
3. Add rest of the ingredients into a bowl and stir. Pour over the cauliflower and stir until well coated.
4. Cook for another 5 minutes.
5. Garnish with scallions and serve.

Cheese Spinach Balls

Serves: 4-6

Ingredients:

- 1 ½ pounds spinach leaves
- 1 cup grated mozzarella cheese
- 1 cup bread crumbs or more if required
- 1 onion, finely chopped
- 1 teaspoon chili flakes
- ½ teaspoon salt or to taste
- 1 tablespoon grated garlic
- ½ cup cornstarch
- Oil for brushing

Method:

1. Place a pot with water over medium heat. Bring to a boil. Add spinach and cook until it wilts. Drain and run under cold water to stop cooking. Place in a colander for a few minutes. Add spinach into the blender. Blend until smooth. Transfer into a large mixing bowl.

2. Add rest of the ingredients except cheese and mix until well combined.

3. Divide the mixture into 12-15 equal portions and shape into balls. Flatten the balls, place a little of the cheese in the center and shape into balls.

4. Brush with oil and place in the air fryer basket which is lined with foil. Fry in batches.

5. Air fry in a preheated air fryer at 390°F for 10-15 minutes or until they are crisp.

6. Serve hot with ketchup.

Grilled Brie with Roasted Cherry Tomatoes

Serves: 3-4

Ingredients:

- 1 pint red and yellow cherry tomatoes
- ½ teaspoon balsamic vinegar
- Freshly ground black pepper to taste
- Salt to taste
- 4 ounces brie cheese
- ½ tablespoon olive oil
- ½ tablespoon chopped fresh parsley
- ½ tablespoon chopped fresh basil
- ½ loaf ciabatta or baguette, sliced, toasted
- Balsamic glaze (optional)

Method:

1. Add cherry tomatoes, oil, vinegar, salt and pepper into a bowl and toss. Transfer into the air fryer basket.
2. Air fry in a preheated air fryer at 225° F for about 45 minutes. Shake the basket 2-3 times while frying. Remove from the air fryer and set aside.
3. Place the air fryer grill pan in the air fryer. Brush Brie with olive oil on both the sides. Place the Brie in the grill pan.

4. Grill for 3 minutes. Flip sides and grill the other side. Remove Brie from the air fryer and place on a serving platter. Drizzle balsamic glaze over it. Garnish with basil and parsley.

5. Serve with toasted baguette and roasted cherry tomatoes.

Chickpea Burgers

Serves: 2

Ingredients:

- 2 cups boiled chickpeas
- 1 small onion, minced
- 1 boiled potato, peeled
- 1 green chili, finely chopped
- ½ teaspoon garam masala
- ½ teaspoon ground cumin
- A handful fresh mint leaves, finely chopped
- 1 tablespoon chopped fresh cilantro
- 1 tablespoon tahini paste or to taste
- Salt to taste
- Oil, for brushing
- 2-3 burger buns, to serve
- Toppings of your choice

Method:

1. Mash the boiled peas and potatoes with a potato masher, in a bowl.
2. Mix in onion, fresh herbs, chili and spices. Add tahini and mix well.
3. Make 2-3 equal portions of the mixture and shape into large patties. Brush with oil. Place in the air fryer basket.

4. Grill in a preheated air fryer at 300° F for 25 minutes. Flip sides half way through grilling.

5. To serve: Split the burgers. Lightly toast the burgers if desired. Place chickpea burgers on the bottom part of the burger. Place toppings on top and serve.

Potato Chips with Sour Cream and Onion Dip

Serves: 1

Ingredients:

- 1 large potato, rinsed, unpeeled, sliced into 1/8 inch thin slices using a slicer
- Freshly ground black pepper to taste

Sour cream and onion dip:

- ½ tablespoon olive oil
- Salt to taste
- Freshly ground pepper to taste
- ¼ cup sour cream
- 1 very small scallion, white parts only, minced
- ½ teaspoon lemon juice or to taste

Method:

1. Rinse the potatoes under cold water. Soak the potato slices in a bowl of cold water for about 15 minutes. Drain the potatoes and place on a kitchen towel in a single layer to dry.
2. Place the chips in the air fryer basket. Spray with cooking spray.
3. Place the basket in the air fryer.

4. Air fry in a preheated air fryer at 300° F for about 15 - 20 minutes or until crisp. Shake the basket a couple of times while frying

5. When chips are ready, sprinkle salt and pepper.

6. Make the dip as follows: Mix together all the ingredients of the dip in a bowl and whisk well.

7. Serve chips with the dip.

Stuffed Okra

Serves: 4-5

Ingredients:

- 1 pound fresh okra, rinsed, trimmed, pat dried
- ½-1 teaspoon chili powder
- ½ teaspoon turmeric powder
- 1 ½ tablespoons ground coriander
- 1 teaspoon
- 1 teaspoon dry mango powder
- 1 ½ teaspoon chat masala
- 1 ½ teaspoons ground cumin powder
- ¾ cup chickpea flour or garbanzo flour
- ½ teaspoon salt
- 1 ½ tablespoons lime juice
- 1 tablespoon vegetable oil

Method:

1. Slit the okra in the middle, horizontally half way through. The area on both the sides should be intact.
2. Mix together, chickpea flour, turmeric powder, chili powder, coriander, cumin, salt and dry mango powder.
3. Add lime juice and ½ tablespoon oil and mix well to make a thick paste.
4. Fill this paste inside each of the okras.

5. Place the stuffed okras in the air fryer basket. Air fry in batches.
6. Air fry in a preheated air fryer at 350° F for 7 minutes.
7. Remove from the air fryer and place on a serving platter.
8. Sprinkle chat masala on top and serve.

Conclusion

I want to thank you once again for choosing this book.

What do you do when you start craving for some French Fries? Do you head out to your favorite fast food outlet? Well, you don't have to do this anymore. You can whip up the perfect French fries at home using an Air Fryer. What's more? You barely need to use any oil to attain perfectly golden and crispy fries!

By now, you might have realized the versatility of the Air Fryer. It indeed is a multipurpose equipment and please don't let its name fool you. This kitchen appliance has clearly revolutionized the way fried food is cooked. You no longer need a vat of fat or oil to fry foods. You can either brush or spray a couple of drops onto the surface of items you wish to fry. Once you do this, you need to sit back and relax and watch as the Air Fryer works its magic. You no longer have to feel guilty about indulging your fried food cravings.

It indeed is a smart investment that is worth every penny you spent. By now, I am certain that you are aware of the simple fact that you don't have to restrict the usage of an Air Fryer to merely frying food and can instead use it to cook different recipes that call for various cooking techniques.

All the recipes that are given in this book are simple to understand and easy to follow. There are hundred Air Fryerfriendly recipes given in this book! By following the recipes given within, you will be able to whip up delicious food like a gourmet chef within no time. Once you get a hang of the different ways in which you can use an Air Fryer, you can experiment with different ingredients to come up with recipes on your own. Try experimenting with different flavors and textures to create healthy and tasty food. The next time you have friends or family over for a watching a match or even for game night, you can certainly blow them away by presenting healthy and tasty fried food!

Finally, if you enjoyed this book, then I'd like to ask you for a favor, would you be kind enough to leave a review for this book on Amazon? It'd be greatly appreciated!

Thank you and good luck!